# PLEASE LEAVE THE SEAT UP
*CONFRONTING MY PROSTATE CANCER WITH HUMOUR*

BRIAN TURNER

*Best Wishes*

*+*

*Good Health*

*Brian Turner*

**TRAFFORD**
PUBLISHING

© Copyright 2006 Brian Turner.
All rights reserved. No part of this publication may be reproduced, stored in
a retrieval system, or transmitted, in any form or by any means, electronic,
mechanical, photocopying, recording, or otherwise, without the written prior
permission of the author.

Note for Librarians: A cataloguing record for this book is available from Library
and Archives Canada at www.collectionscanada.ca/amicus/index-e.html

ISBN 1-4120-9529-8

*Printed in Victoria, BC, Canada. Printed on paper with minimum 30% recycled fibre.
Trafford's print shop runs on "green energy" from solar, wind and other environmentally-friendly
power sources.*

**TRAFFORD**
PUBLISHING™

*Offices in Canada, USA, Ireland and UK*

**Book sales for North America and international:**
Trafford Publishing, 6E–2333 Government St.,
Victoria, BC V8T 4P4 CANADA
phone 250 383 6864 (toll-free 1 888 232 4444)
fax 250 383 6804; email to orders@trafford.com

**Book sales in Europe:**
Trafford Publishing (UK) Limited, 9 Park End Street, 2nd Floor
Oxford, UK OX1 1HH UNITED KINGDOM
phone +44 (0)1865 722 113 (local rate 0845 230 9601)
facsimile +44 (0)1865 722 868; info.uk@trafford.com

**Order online at:**
trafford.com/06-1284

10 9 8 7 6 5 4 3 2

To my wife Carol who suffered so much more than I did in the darkest days of 'our' cancer but whose support and love has never faltered, despite having to deal with her own crisis of homesickness and isolation.

# Acknowledgements

I would like to thank my boss, Kevin Ball, for first suggesting that I had a story worth telling. Without his provocation and encouragement, I would never have put pen to paper. When I did get started on the book, even before I had the bare bones of the story, I sought the help of my sister, Betty Keen. Throughout the time it took me to write, she spent many tireless hours reading and correcting my script. Her help and guidance has been invaluable.

An enormous debt of gratitude goes to all the doctors, nurses and medical staff in America for their dedication to get me through the nine months of treatment. My biggest thanks go to Doctor Friedman whose straight talking and dogged determination to beat the cancer helped me to have the same attitude in coping with it.

The book, by necessity, contains quite a lot of detailed information and much of it was researched on the Internet, although the information on the disease and the various treatments came from my urologists' handouts. However, by far the most useful source of information came from a book by Desiree Lyon Howe entitled *His Prostate and Me*. Her book was compelling reading for me immediately after my operation, although, with hindsight, it would have been better if I had read it beforehand. I would recommend this book to anyone who is suffering from prostate cancer.

*Brian Turner*

So many people have given me support and encouragement throughout. They probably don't know how much they have helped, but by being there for me and keeping in touch, I found the strength to keep going. Although I am bound to miss a few for which I apologise. These include Peter Duffy and Phil Piddington, who were both former bosses of mine. They rang me often to provide support. Ian Smith has been a true friend in every respect and his help, both supportive and practical, has allowed me to keep my sanity. My colleagues in America, Mark Proegler, Andy Donaghue and Mike Rudd, who, together with their respective wives, Amy, Katy and Karen, have been an important part of my support system. Others include Lesley Rubie and Mike Hammock, John and Judith Edwards, Sarah and Terry Williams and the many friends and work colleagues who all helped in so many ways.

Several people assisted me by reviewing the book and highlighting mistakes and omissions and suggesting changes and refinements. The major input came from John Bromwich and Niall Enright although a great many others helped with their constructive critique. Thank you all for tirelessly plodding through the early drafts in order to help hone the book into shape.

Finally, I would like to say a special thank you to our dear friends Jason Rundle and his wife Karen, whose offers of help were unremitting. Their daughter Olivia was born the day before my operation and it has been an inspiration to me to watch her grow and develop, sharing the same goals with our potty training.

# Contents

Acknowledgements . . . . . . . . . . . . . . . . . . . . 5
Introduction . . . . . . . . . . . . . . . . . . . . . . . 9
1. Welcome to America . . . . . . . . . . . . . 13
2. Discoveries . . . . . . . . . . . . . . . . . . . 21
3. Education Required . . . . . . . . . . . . . . 29
4. Making Choices . . . . . . . . . . . . . . . . 40
5. 'What's up Doc'? . . . . . . . . . . . . . . . . 50
6. Gleason Revealed . . . . . . . . . . . . . . . 61
7. Sharing the News . . . . . . . . . . . . . . . 69
8. Preparing for the Chop . . . . . . . . . . . . 80
9. The Final Cut . . . . . . . . . . . . . . . . . . 91
10. Good to be Home . . . . . . . . . . . . . . . 105
11. Messing with my Hormones . . . . . . . . 120
12. Them Bones, Them Bones . . . . . . . . . 128
13. Paget's or Cancer. That is the Question . . . 135
14. Eradication . . . . . . . . . . . . . . . . . . 145
15. 'Ow's it Going? . . . . . . . . . . . . . . . . 151
16. The Last Word . . . . . . . . . . . . . . . . 162
Appendix A . . . . . . . . . . . . . . . . . . . . 163
Appendix B . . . . . . . . . . . . . . . . . . . . 164
Appendix C . . . . . . . . . . . . . . . . . . . . 166
Appendix D . . . . . . . . . . . . . . . . . . . . 168

## Introduction

**I** have always had a positive disposition and the ability to look on the bright side of life. In the days and weeks that passed following the diagnosis of prostate cancer, I spent many hours talking with friends and colleagues: either they would phone or call in person to enquire about my progress. Although cancer is an extremely serious matter, there were many events along the way that I found amusing and I would often regale them with my stories and snippets of conversations I'd had with this or that doctor, and we would laugh together.

As I worked my way through the treatment, many difficult and potentially upsetting times occurred where I really needed my friends and relied on their conversation and support. Throughout that time, I always took the most optimistic view of things, either through blind ignorance or an unmitigated determination not to allow myself to become a statistic on the role of cancer victims. Many times in the past my mind had wandered to thinking how I might finally turn up my toes, giving up my fight against immortality, but to die of cancer was never on my agenda. Not then and not now.

About three months after my operation, I was having dinner with my boss in a particularly good Italian restaurant in Houston Texas. It was a difficult time as the doctors had just advised me that the cancer had spread to my pelvis. Over dinner I shared some of my stories and he found himself laughing out loud several times at amusing events about my time at the hospital or the mechanics of dealing with the side effects of the treatment. He suddenly realised that he was laughing and apologised for apparently finding my current predicament so amusing. He said, "It must be pretty awful for you right now, but you do seem to have the ability to make it all sound so funny." His comment was a real tonic to me. I hadn't particularly set out to amuse him, but it meant that I'd managed to hold onto the one vital attribute which has carried me well through my life and through the good, the bad and the downright awful aspects of my cancer: A good sense of humour.

As we were leaving the restaurant after an excellent dinner and an enjoyable evening of banter, Kevin said, "I have never heard anyone talk about cancer in such a blunt and light-hearted way – you ought to write a book." I dismissed the notion on the spot, thinking that the sooner I could put all this behind me, the better. However, a week or two later, in a reflective moment, I decided that I should commit my experience to paper. I felt it would help me get the whole thing in a better perspective and really understand all the events, many of which at the time had seemed like a blur. I often felt that I'd been carried along by events, without truly understanding what was going on, or why.

As I shaped the story in my mind, I realised that there had been many times when I had struggled with problems associated with the treatment, before eventually finding a solution and thinking if only I could speak to someone who has gone through this, it would make life a lot easier for me. I have therefore tried to write this, not only as a story, but also with information and tips, which I have learned along the way. Hopefully, some men (and their partners) will gain a clearer understanding about the function of the prostate so they are better prepared to recognise if out-of-the ordinary situations occur, and be able to deal with them in a timely manner when things start to go wrong. I hope that a little of my experience may help people who either have to face up to the disease personally or who want to help others through their own battle, to deal with some of the more practical issues. In my attempt to cater for all groups of reader, I am aware that a few chapters, from necessity, deal with medical issues in quite a lot of detail. However, this detail will be essential for anyone suffering with prostate cancer but may be of less interest to the casual reader. Whatever your reason for reading my book, I hope you will find many of the events amusing and that you will smile along with me.

# 1
# Welcome to America

"We'll open you up and take a sample from your lymph nodes, and keep you comfortable while we get the analysis from the lab. If it's clear, we'll carry on and remove your prostate. However, if we find traces of cancer beyond the prostate, we'll just sew you up and send you home."

Doctor Freidman, the urologist overseeing the radical removal of my prostate, was giving my wife and me a final briefing, only minutes before I was wheeled into the operating theatre. This news came as a bombshell to me and I could only imagine what terror it now struck in Carol's already tortured mind. For me, it was confirmation that this was pretty serious. Until now I had thought, only a short stay in hospital while they cut out the offending gland, then back to work after the Christmas break. The news, which the doctor had just announced, made me think that my expectations and overall grasp of exactly how serious this was had been a little unrealistic. For Carol this was the worst possible news. She'd been to hell and back in her mind, since I was first diagnosed with cancer six weeks earlier: She was already viewing the rest of my life with a dismal sense of foreboding and wondering when the Almighty was going to carry me off. The doctor's latest comment was now playing to her worst fears. Maybe the tumour was more widespread than we thought and I was doomed to the inevitable road of terminal cancer. In her mind, this would now only be a matter of time.

Although I was really concerned about Carol's state of mind, right now, I had neither the time, nor the inclination to dwell on her, or on the doctor's comments. I'd already had my pre-med and in a few moments, would be unconscious by the expert hands of the anaesthetist. After that, events would run their course and I could do all my worrying when I woke up. Carol, on the other hand, had three and a half agonizing hours to wait, until she would learn the outcome.

---

With my weight edging towards 18 stones and being only 5'8" tall, I cast a wide shadow and have always felt that a good diet was way overdue, although this did nothing to detract from my jolly disposition. I have enjoyed good health throughout my life and although I can't profess to having never been ill, I have only really had the usual coughs and colds, which do the rounds each winter. Good fortune has shone on me to the extent that I have avoided anything even slightly serious. My only bouts in hospital were when I had my appendix out at the age of fourteen and for a couple of days back in the mid nineties when I had a stone passing through my kidneys. Well, the doctor said it was a stone but judging by the pain as it landed in the urinal, I'm convinced it was a house brick.

With such rude health, life was generally good and as I have always been able to laugh in the face of adversity, I tried to ensure that I helped those around me to do the same. In the middle of 2001 I had just passed my 50th birthday and more than a few grey hairs had dared to infiltrate the mop of dark curls, which I had been blessed with as a boy. My hairdresser kindly described it as a 'distinguished' salt and pepper look, but I couldn't help thinking that it was a sign of my advancing years. I didn't feel that I was old yet but I realised that I was more than halfway through my life, which made me determined to use the time I had left, to the full.

I was expecting my work in Energy Management with a multinational company to see me through to the end of my working life. I'd often considered a move from the part of the business which I had worked in for 17 years, but I'd been extremely fortunate and felt quite privileged to have helped shape it during my time with them. Joining as a technician in 1986, I'd worked my way through the ranks until I became the head of the Operations team only 12 years later. I was now a senior manager and, with responsibility for over 300 staff, was clearly an influential member of the management team. I enjoyed the status of elder statesman, given that I was now the longest serving person in the company, and welcomed the many calls on my time for my perspective on various issues, often far outside my own area of responsibility. In short, I felt that I had arrived - and no one was snapping at my heels to replace me. The post was mine until I decided to vacate the chair.

My job was to direct and control a team of middle and junior managers, coordinating teams of blue-collar workers at customer sites, managing their utilities plant and moreover, their energy requirements. The customers were typically the household names of car manufacturers, food and confectionery producers and the like.

But primarily, they all had energy bills of at least half a million pounds per annum. With the recent introduction of a government levy on companies for the energy they used, energy management had come into sharp focus for our commercial and industrial customers, at least one of which faced levy charges in excess of a million pounds a year. It wasn't complacency that caused my feeling of contentment in my job; I knew I was at the top of my own little tree and this new focus on energy created an environment, which would occupy us all for many years to come. It would certainly be enough to see me through to the end of my working life.

Away from work, Carol and I enjoyed foreign travel and went abroad whenever we could. During our holidays we'd visited over thirty countries on four continents during our 22 years of marriage. We'd often discussed how wonderful it would be to have the opportunity of living abroad for a few years and at times during my career this did look possible. However, with us both now in our fifties we were thinking more about our plans for retirement than uprooting ourselves. It therefore came as a surprise to me and a shock to Carol, when Kevin, a former colleague who was now heading up a new "Group Energy Enhancement" initiative, rung to ask if I would be interested in leading an internal energy programme, similar to the one we had been running with external customers for many years. He told me that it would most likely involve a two-to-three-year stint in America, which obviously implied that we would need to up sticks and move house for the duration.

Maybe it shouldn't have been such a surprise. It

seemed that most of my colleagues and those who knew me best thought that I'd be an ideal person to drive the initiative, working on the ground, particularly in America. Our American business accounted for nearly 80% of all the energy the company used: in excess of a billion dollars a year. I'd taken on and conquered many challenges in my current role over the years and I realised that if I wanted another big challenge before I finally went off to spend more time with my family, this was probably it.

After a lot of soul-searching, cajoling and arm-twisting, Carol agreed to support me on this venture. That was no real surprise, as she always supported anything I'd taken on at work and sacrificed a major part of her social life in order to do so. But this was different. This wasn't simply another house move to a place where she knew no one: this was to a different country in a different continent. I really needed her to be comfortable with it. Reflecting back on our various travel adventures and the knowledge we'd gained by experiencing such rich and diverse cultures as India, East Africa, Romania and Hungary, we believed that we would benefit from the wider experience of living and immersing ourselves in yet another culture. Besides, with the exception of a short cruise around the West Indies, calling in at St Thomas, and Carol's brief shopping trip to New York a few years earlier, America had avoided our attention so far and we needed to put that right.

As we had few ties there was really nothing standing in our way, we decided to give it a try. The next day I gave Kevin the green light to put plans in place.

I started the new job in November 2001, although it would be ten months before I eventually set up home in the US and for Carol, it would be a further six weeks after that. During the first half of 2002 British Airways were "taking more care of me" or more to the point, taking more fare from me, as I spent much of my time flying between London and Washington State or Texas. However, in July 2002 we finally packed up our home in the UK and saw it whisked away in a shipping container, hoping that we would soon be re-united with it in our new home in Houston.

In early August 2002 I said goodbye to all my friends and family and made my final preparations for our move to the US. Carol was now living in a flat at the place where she worked, with only a bed and a few sticks of furniture, which she would eventually dispose of before following me out. On 12th August she took me to the airport for my flight to Houston. We were full of hope and looking forward to our new adventure, although the six weeks apart was not something we were delighted about – but it was necessary. Carol had to work through her notice period and a number of loose ends still remained to be attended to. However, as she waved me off that morning, neither of us had any inkling of the events which would start to unfold for me in America - even before she left the shores of the UK.

Houston is one of the five largest cities in America and home to over five million people. It is in south Texas about 60 miles from the Gulf of Mexico. Its growth from a small town to a major city was due to one thing. Oil! And it was the oil business that had brought me here. However, since the early sixties Houston has had a second and more exciting claim to fame. The Johnson Space Centre in South Houston is home to NASA's mission control, and has been the control centre for all American space flight since it opened, throughout the Mercury, Gemini, Apollo and Shuttle programmes. Today, it is also the control centre for the International Space Station.

'Houston' was actually the first word to be spoken on the moon. In July 1969 Neil Armstrong sent goose bumps around the world when he calmly announced "Houston, Tranquillity base here. The Eagle has landed". With that kind of auspicious history to fire my enthusiasm, I knew I was going to enjoy living and working in the city. It set the tone and the closeness of this living history was an inspiration to me.

At 6.30 on my first full day in America I was at my desk in my new office, keen to get started and already making arrangements to meet people and visit the company's sites in order to start things moving on the energy front. At least being on my own for a while meant that I could concentrate on work and not worry about what time I got home each evening. I had a lot to do and I wanted to make an immediate impact on the job. For the first month I'd rented a furnished apartment and with the exception of buying food and drink, and learning how to cook, life had little to slow me down in those first few weeks. That is, with the exception of the administration of establishing oneself in a new land. I doubt if America is worse than any other country but wading through the paperwork and bureaucracy was a pile of grief I hadn't anticipated.

After a few weeks of working through and overcoming the problems of obtaining a social security number, setting up a bank account in order that I could be paid, and taking the Texan state driving test, the final piece of admin was to get myself registered with a GP or Primary Care Physician (PCP) as they call them in the US. Even that was not without its problems as not all PCPs were available to me. I discovered that it would depend on the Insurance Company I was registered with, and when I looked on the insurance web site for PCPs in my area, I came across dozens. I was struggling to decide how best to choose. Picking the nearest surgery sounded sensible but I had no knowledge of the system. Luckily a colleague was on hand to advise me and after a short discussion, recommend his own PCP, whom he found "user friendly." This sounded perfect and I booked an immediate appointment, as I needed to get a prescription for my ongoing medication requirements for high blood pressure and cholesterol. I'd had the foresight to bring a month's supply of medication with me but obviously I didn't want to run out of pills before I could see the doctor. As I was unaware of the system for obtaining medication, but suspecting it to be similarly bogged down in red tape as my earlier experiences had been, I wanted to allow a reasonable period of safety between my requirements and the time when I could be seen by the PCP. I made an appointment for 5th September.

# 2
# Discoveries

As I waited in Doctor Epstein's office that day, I was unprepared for the events that unfolded, quite unlike any previous visit I'd made to a doctor in the past. I sat in the plush waiting room and watched the news on the TV in the corner. I could have made use of the free telephone except, as yet, I hardly knew anyone to call. At the allotted time I was shown into the doctor's office, where I was weighed and screened by his nurse. Very soon an intern came in and questioned me about my previous medical history. I think this was as much for his training as it was to do with my medical needs, as the PCP repeated the process when we eventually met.

Doctor Epstein was a warm, friendly guy with a firm handshake. From the moment I met him I felt at ease and we quickly got into a conversation about 'me'. Not from a medical perspective but my reason for being in the US, my general interests and where I would be living. For the next fifteen minutes he told me where the good local restaurants were and some general points about things to do in Houston. All useful stuff but not what I'd expected from him. My previous experience with GPs was that I had just enough time to sit down, stick my tongue out and say "aarhh!" before he thrust a prescription in my hand and I found myself outside the door again. But not Doctor Epstein: he was making me feel like a valued customer already and we'd only just met. He asked me once more to go over my medical history, but this time in more detail. When he learned that I was suffering from hypertension (high blood pressure) and high cholesterol, he said, "You're my kind of patient. We're going to have fun working together." It appeared that, by accident, I'd had the good fortune to register with a doctor who specialized in the very conditions that had troubled me for over ten years. Serendipity or what? He was already talking about working to overcome these rather than spending a lifetime of treatment with drugs. This was exactly what I had wanted from a doctor for many years and had failed to get one interested in anything beyond leaving repeat prescriptions with the receptionist, thereby avoiding seeing me to discuss a longer-term approach.

As we came close to the end of our session, Doctor Epstein wrote me a prescription for the American equivalent of the medication I was using. As an aside, he mentioned that in the US it was usual to screen men over 50 for prostate and colon cancer. He asked if I'd had any screening recently and I confirmed that this type of screening wasn't the current practice in the UK. He asked my permission to carry out Digital Rectal Examination or DRE, as I now affectionately know them. I was impressed. I knew that medical advances in the US were way ahead of those in the UK but I hadn't even heard of a digital rectal examination. I couldn't help thinking that far from using this approach back home; we probably didn't even have the technology to carry out analogue rectal examinations yet. I was trying to imagine what such a high-tech piece of equipment would look like and awaited his next move, keen to see this recent space-age innovation.

## Please Leave The Seat Up

Doctor Epstein started to slide a pair of rubber gloves onto his hands, and said with a wry smile, "In these circumstances, it pays to choose your PCP carefully. Look!" he held up his right arm, "small hands." Realisation hit me all at once: What I'd imagined as being high tech was actually very low tech. The 'Digital' in DRE related to 'digit'. I hadn't realised when I left home that day, that I would become so intimately familiar with the doctor, but here I was lying across his examination couch, while he carried out 'the screening' with his gloved hand. It's hard to take much in when you have a finger firmly probing your rectum but I was aware of him musing out loud as he poked and prodded around. Standing upright and allowing me to pull up my trousers, he said with no particular emphasis, "Mmmmm, well your prostate feels a slightly unusual shape. It's probably nothing but I'm going to ask you to have a PSA test all the same." He invited me to step across the hall to the lab before I left the surgery. I did as I was asked and the nurse drew a sample of my blood and I went on my merry way.

As I thought back to this first meeting with my PCP, my only recollection of the visit was his friendly approach and my need to rush home and write down the names of all the restaurants he'd suggested, in case I forgot and had to forgo the gastronomic pleasures he had so eagerly discussed with me. I certainly didn't have any lasting thoughts regarding my DRE; or the blood test, which followed.

A few days later I was just getting out of my car to go into Starbucks for a tall Latte when my mobile rang.

## Brian Turner

"Hi, Mr. Turner, this is Roger Epstein. Remember the PSA we did the other day? Well it's come back a bit on the high side and I wanted to just check it one more time. Can you swing by my office when it's convenient and we'll draw a little more blood, if that's OK with you?"

Of course it was OK with me. He was the doctor and if he needed another test, who was I to argue. His casual attitude gave no suggestion of concern or urgency so a little later, after I'd sat outside Starbucks, enjoying the sun, my hot coffee and an oatmeal and raisin cookie, I was back at the lab giving another armful of blood. Doctor Epstein suggested I called in on Monday to discuss the results.

---

Bang on time Roger called me in and shared his thoughts with me regarding the two PSA tests. He told me that they were higher than he would have expected at 2.9 and 3.6 respectively, but he wouldn't normally be inclined to take any further action unless it was over 4. "However," he said, "I'm going to make an exception in your case because it doesn't 'feel' quite right to me. And I'm also curious as to why the PSA appears to have increased by over 0.5 in a few days. It could just be that one of the tests was wrong but I'm gonna suggest that you go and see Doctor Nash. He's an excellent urologist."

Once again I was happy to oblige and acceded to the nice doctor's request. In my book, anyone who could make recommendations of so many excellent restaurants was obviously a man of good judgment and someone to be trusted. I felt sure he knew what he was talking about, and anyway, I had no idea what a PSA test was, nor for that matter, what an urologist did for a living. But if Doctor Epstein said to go and see him, I wasn't going to argue. I rang Doctor Nash's office and made an appointment for 30th September then put it out of my mind. After all, that was a few weeks away and I still had so much to do before Carol arrived.

I had just moved out of my temporary apartment and into our rented house, which over the next few weeks I needed to turn into a home. The furniture arrived intact, having survived the nearly 5000-mile trip across the Atlantic and the removal guys worked in temperatures well over 100 degrees to shift it all into place. By the end of the day they looked a little hot, but even though I'd only watched and directed operations, I was like a soggy dishrag. How they managed to work in the heat I will never know.

By the time I returned to the UK to escort Carol back to the US, everything was in place and looking cosy. During the process, one of the most immediate problems I'd encountered was the recognition that the electrical voltages, telephones and TV broadcast formats are incompatible between the two countries, rendering almost all our electrical equipment completely useless for the duration of our stay. I indulged in an orgy of spending for the first few weeks, to ensure that all the creature comforts were in place ahead of Carol's arrival. Without a doubt, the 'buying' experience in the

US is completely different to that in the UK. Firstly, electrical goods are significantly cheaper and the shops compete vigorously for your dollars. I remember when I purchased a TV at an amazingly low price; I was very surprised to find that it came with a free leather swivel chair. I installed them both in the new house about a week before our furniture arrived. The TV sat in one corner of the large lounge and the chair took centre place. Although the rest of the house was completely empty, I couldn't help thinking to myself that we now had all the creature comforts we needed – and all for the price of a TV.

More importantly, I also needed to purchase two cars, as the public transport system in Houston is non-existent and without your own transport you can't even leave the house: especially in Houston's extremely hot weather, where walking is well nigh impossible. Buying a car in the US was one of the experiences I really enjoyed. I was fascinated that I could wander in off the street at seven o clock in the evening, test drive a car then negotiate until I got the price to where I wanted it, and be able to drive out with it by eight-thirty the same evening. I knew that if the negotiation had been more protracted, the salesman would have been happy to stay until he concluded a deal – even if it was past midnight. That was reinforced when I purchased the second car, where the salesman and I were still locked in battle at nine-thirty. And yes, I did get the deal I wanted and yes; I did drive the car home that night.

My manic spending in order to get things in place before Carol's arrival had clearly come to the attention of some friends. One of them, Karen, who had witnessed my arrival home each day, laden with new gadgets, casually asked, "When are you going to stop spending?" I was having a ball but knew it couldn't last. I gave my game away when I had to admit that it would stop as soon as Carol arrived. That day was close at hand and on 24th September I boarded the British Airways 2024 flight with great excitement, bringing our six-week separation to an end. I arrived at Carol's flat at about 8.30 a.m. on the morning of 25th which just also happened to be her birthday, making the reunion even more special. We were so thrilled to be together again, although Carol would go through a traumatic few days before we could leave the shores for our new home.

Adjusting to a new lifestyle was not too difficult for me. I was staying with the same company and working with people I had got to know quite well over the last year. This was simply a change of country with a much warmer climate in the Gulf of Mexico, where, even in the winter, temperatures rarely fall below 15 degrees Celsius. And America is *the* consumer society, for which I was ideally suited. I couldn't imagine how anyone could fail to enjoy it. For Carol her feelings were entirely different. Not only was she moving house to a new and unfamiliar country, she was also at the end of her working life and wouldn't be taking on a job in the US (her visa didn't allow it, even if she wanted to). She was retiring from a career she had loved and one which she excelled at. For the last seven and a half years she had been the manager of a Sheltered Housing Scheme for the elderly. She not only did the job extremely well, but far exceeded what was expected of her. In the period she had been in the post, she had helped the residents raise considerable funds through various sales and functions, enabling them to have parties, outings, holidays and other events throughout the year. Moreover, they had been able to construct a fabulous garden, which only the week before she was to leave, had won first prize in the borough's Garden in Bloom competition. Everyone knew she would be a hard act to follow: her bosses had told her as much. But the residents didn't want her to leave – ever!

Clearly, breaking this relationship was going to be as difficult for her as it was for the residents, which is why I'd agreed to fly back to the UK and be with her for her leaving party. We all knew it was going to be an emotional event, but when the time came, Carol was so overwhelmed that she couldn't deliver her leaving speech. I agreed to do it on her behalf, but it proved to be a harrowing experience for everyone, with many people openly weeping throughout the whole time. I had anticipated that it would be difficult and was concerned that Carol would find it so hard to say her goodbyes. We had agreed that after the speeches, we would make our excuses and leave, rather than stay around, prolonging the tears for everyone. Even so, it was a traumatic time for Carol and she was not in a good frame of mind for the start of our new adventure as our plane took off from Gatwick at 10 a.m. the next morning.

# 3
# Education Required

I knew everything I needed to know about the prostate. It was a bit like the appendix, right? No useful function but if it became enlarged, it made you pee a lot. This condition was mostly associated with old men who sat around all day in nursing homes, smelling of urine.

For those as poorly educated on these medical matters as me, the prostate is not at all like the appendix and clearly has two important functions, of which I would be made painfully aware later, but for now I simply wanted to know a bit more about PSA and the dreaded DRE.

To avoid any errors, I have not tried to relay this in my own words but chosen instead to quote from two excellent works, which I came across in my bid to become more informed. This insight was the first step on my road to education of all things 'prostate'.

With regard to examinations for early detection of prostate cancer, the recommendations of the American Urological Association are as follows:

*"Annual **digital rectal examination** (DRE) and serum **prostate specific antigen** (PSA) measurement substantially increase the early detection of prostate cancer. These tests are most appropriate for male patients 50 years of age or older and for those 40 or older who are high risk, including those of African-American de-*

*scent and those with a family history of prostate cancer. Patients in these age and risk groups should be given the option to participate in screening or early detection programs. PSA testing should continue in a healthy male who has a life expectancy of ten or more years."*

The American Cancer Society Prostate Cancer Screening guidelines similarly state:

*"Beginning at age 50, all men who have at least a 10-year life expectancy should be offered both the PSA blood test and a digital rectal exam. Men in high-risk groups, such as African Americans, men with close family members (fathers, brothers or sons) who have had prostate cancer diagnosed at a young age should begin testing at 45 years.*

*"The blood test used in the screening process, measures the level of specific protein in the blood, prostatic specific antigens (PSA), which is generated by prostatic tissue and is used to help detect prostate cancer. PSA is a prostate specific test not a cancer specific test. Therefore, a higher than normal PSA does not necessarily indicate cancer, it indicates the presence of prostatic disease, prostate enlargement, infection or prostate cancer. However, as cancerous prostate tissue secretes approximately 10 times as much PSA as normal tissue, it is a good indicator of prostate cancer, particularly at higher levels or if the reading is increasing quickly.*

*"Most of the PSA is located in the small tubes, which store semen that runs throughout the prostate.*

*However, small amounts leak into the bloodstream and can be measured with the PSA blood test. The likelihood of a man having prostate cancer increases as the PSA level increases.*

*The normal reference range of PSA is 0-4. When levels of PSA are higher than 4 it can indicate prostate cancer, although further tests are needed to determine the diagnosis. To complicate matters further, a PSA of 4 or less does not necessarily mean that a man is free from prostate cancer, but in most instances the medical profession uses the benchmark of 4 and above to determine when further tests may be necessary. A PSA between 4 and 10 does not automatically indicate prostate cancer, but it will trigger the requirement for additional tests as it indicates a 30% risk that prostate cancer will be present. A PSA above 10 is more likely to indicate clinical prostate cancer and will almost always result in a biopsy.*

*"The screening process is to test the PSA level annually and note any change. Using this method, doctors can detect a potential cancer or a reoccurrence of the disease following treatment. If the PSA is above the reference point of 0-4 or it has been escalating more than ¾ of a point in a year, an examination by an Urologist is recommended in order to determine the specific reason for the elevation.*

Having read and understood all that, I was now clearer about the need to see the urologist. Obviously, with a PSA of less than four, I was happy to note that at the very worst, the swelling in my prostate was a minor issue and even if it were found to be cancerous in nature, it was likely to be in the early stages and could be dealt with quite easily. My trip to see Doctor Nash was clearly precautionary rather than due to any real concern at this stage. Well, that was my take on it anyway.

My appointment with Doctor Nash was scheduled for 30th September, only 3 days after Carol and I had arrived back from the UK. On arrival at the doctor's office I was given a pile of forms to fill in. In fact, his nurse had called me the day before, to ask if I could come in 30 minutes ahead of my appointment time, in order to wade through the form filling. Apart from the usual stuff about medical history and general information: age, sex, height, weight, I was given a big checklist regarding bladder activity, none of which I'd thought about before but happily indulged in. A bit like one of those 20-question things they often have in magazines to determine if you are a hot lover, a good husband, or a chocoholic. I was asked to tick the boxes if I experienced any of the following:

- A need to urinate frequently
- A problem stopping or starting urination
- Hesitancy or difficulty in starting urination
- A feeling that the bladder has not emptied after urination
- An interrupted or weaker than normal urine flow
- Inability to urinate in spite of the pressure to do so
- Pain or a burning sensation during urination
- Nocturia (waking up in the night to urinate)
- Blood in the semen or urine

- Pain in the hips, kidneys, lower back or during ejaculation

As I worked my way down the form, ticking the odd box here and there, I stopped thinking about whether my score would show me as a true romantic and found myself thinking instead, well, at least I'm starting to understand what an urologist does for a living. I couldn't help reflecting that his type of work would be way down in my list of 'interesting ways to spend the day at the office'. I even went so far as to think that someone was taking the p... but pulled myself up, reminding myself that someone had to do these things, I was just glad it wasn't me.

Doctor Nash was a tall, grey-haired guy in his mid-fifties. He was in good shape and obviously worked out a fair bit. He had an excellent bedside manner and discussed why it was necessary to heed the signs from my previous PSA and DRE examinations. He then beamed a wide smile and said, "Most people shake hands when they meet, however, as I'm an urologist I'll just ask you to drop your trousers and bend over." An interesting approach but I got his drift and slipped my trousers and pants down around my ankles. This was starting to become a habit, and not one I wanted to repeat too often. As it turned out, it was a habit that was to become second nature to me over the next few months.

Doctor Nash, who, thankfully, also had fairly small hands, carried out his DRE examination. He seemed to be much more thorough than Doctor Epstein, but then this was his area of expertise – his specialist subject if you like. This only reinforced my earlier thoughts about the unattractiveness of his chosen profession and why anyone with a free choice, would elect to do it. He started to prod and poke; each movement punctuated with a knowing "Hhhumm!" After poking around for considerably longer than I was happy with, he asked me to get dressed again and we sat back down. He confirmed Doctor Epstein's previous thoughts that the prostate was misshapen, adding that he was concerned enough by his findings to want to investigate further into the reason for the swelling. He told me that he wasn't worried at this stage and he urged me not to worry either. He was preaching to the converted. I wasn't worried, nor had I been during this whole process. In fact, the only worry I had now was that he had told me not to worry. Why did he think I would? I assured him that I was totally relaxed about it all and would only be concerned if he told me there was something to be concerned about. He smiled and asked that I have yet another PSA. Why not, I thought, at this rate the US medical profession will have more of my blood in test tubes than I have left in my veins. Again, I was off down the hall to roll up my sleeve for the lab nurse.

A few days later the doctor called to advise me that the PSA was 3.8. That pleased me, as it was still below 4, which the experts seem to think is a magic number, so this was good news as far as I was concerned; more of an annoyance than a problem. Doctor Nash asked me to book in with him so that he could have a proper look with an ultrasound. I accepted that this was how it was going to be. More and more tests, until the doctors had satisfied themselves that I was OK. I was simply going along for the ride.

I was my normal relaxed self as I arrived for the ultrasound examination. Carol had accompanied me to Doctor Nash's office, not for any particular reason although I think she felt that I might be glad of company. She had only been in the US for three weeks and was still having trouble finding her way around, so her reasons for coming were as much for her education on the geographic layout of Houston as they were for my company. She waited in the outer office when I went through for my examination.

I had no idea what the ultrasound would be like. I'd had one before on my leg and obviously was aware of their use for pregnant women. However, I was curious as to what area of my body he would need to draw the sensor across, in order to see my prostate. As I entered the examination room, this mystery was removed in short order. Hanging beside the screen was the sensor, which looked remarkably like a penis; only it had a long handle on it. This was not at all what I had in mind. I tend to try not to think about medical procedures ahead of time, as it's usually nowhere near as bad as the picture your mind conjures up. However, on this occasion I was wrong: the ultrasound[1] was going to be every bit as bad, and then some. I was thankful that I hadn't spent time imagining it and I simply wanted it over and done with now. Doctor Nash, ever mindful of the need for customer's service, didn't delay the process a moment

---

[1] *To use its proper name, Transrectal ultrasonography (or TRUS) is a process where sound waves that cannot be heard by humans (ultrasound) are sent out by a probe inserted in the rectum. The waves bounce off the prostate, and a computer uses the echoes to create a picture called a sonogram.*

longer than necessary. He asked me remove my trousers and pants and lie on the examination table with my knees drawn up to my stomach in a foetal position (or was it a fatal position)? He lost no time in lubricating the sensor, before inserting the beast deftly into my rectum. This could have been a moment when homophobia started to kick in, in a big way, but it suddenly struck me that this was potentially quite serious. For the first time since I dropped my trousers in Doctor Epstein's office, I realised that things had moved to a stage where time, effort and significant amounts of money were now being invested in trying to establish what was happening to cause my prostate to have become enlarged and misshapen. Whatever it was, clearly it wasn't normal and other people were obviously concerned, so maybe it was time for me to show a little concern. Up until now I was so unconcerned that I'd not even discussed it with Carol. I had been quite content for the doctors to do their tests and satisfy themselves that everything was OK.

But then, Doctor Nash gave me the first indication that indeed, things were not OK. In fact, when he said he was going to take some biopsies he had my complete and undivided attention. As I lay there, it was all going around in my head. My PSA was on the increase, I had an enlarged and misshapen prostate, and I was now going to have a biopsy. I had only limited knowledge of the medical business but to me a biopsy meant tumour. As I lay there I concluded that the biopsy was purely to determine whether it was benign or malignant. My thoughts were abruptly interrupted with a sharp pain coming from somewhere inside my rectum as he took his first of six samples.

Given that I hadn't spent much time ahead of the appointment thinking about the problem, it will come as no surprise to learn that I didn't actually know where the prostate was situated in my body, nor for that matter, what its exact function was. More about its function later but right now I was on a voyage of self-discovery of its location. The pain of each extracted sample was enough to direct my attention to its precise position and made me aware of exactly how difficult it is to get at. Curiosity got the better of me sometime later and I discovered that the prostate is located below the bladder and in front of the rectum. Given its position, it is difficult to imagine how a sample of it can be taken via the rectal duct. However, the process is cunningly brilliant, if not somewhat medieval in its application. A spring-loaded needle mounted on the end of the ultrasound sensor is pushed up against the rectal wall. When in position, the needle is sprung. In a flash, it plunges through the wall and into the tissue of the prostate, before springing back out with a sample firmly in its grasp. This is repeated on several areas of the prostate to ensure that a good overall sample is recovered.

Apart from the painful aspect of the process, which I was starting to get used to, the sensation associated with each sample was causing a pretty weird reaction to my organs. By sample number five I was feeling an urgent need to empty my bowels and bladder. I began to fear that at any moment I may not be able to hold on any longer and we would all end up in a big mess. I was so relieved when Doctor Nash said, "OK that's all". He told me to get dressed and he would come back to talk to me when I was ready. Right now all I needed a trip to the bathroom.

We sat across a small table as he started to give me the news. I knew what was coming so I was already prepared, which I think was a relief to him. He looked me squarely in the eyes and said, "We need to wait for the results of the biopsy, but I won't be at all surprised if they reveal that this is a malignant tumour." I watched his body and eye movements. I have always being acutely sensitive of people's non-verbal communications and I detected the truth he was not telling me. This was his way of preparing me for the bad news when it finally came. No need: I was already fully prepared. I have always had the ability to take any news and deal with it rationally and unemotionally, as if it's general information. I have approached things in this way throughout my working life and I have found it a useful method of assimilating information and being able to decide on a plan of action, without the baggage of emotion. I guess for most people this would have been a moment of devastation but for me this was merely another piece of information to be dealt with. I took this news in the same detached way, rather than reacting as if it were something closely associated with my well-being. My immediate and only reaction was to ask about the next steps. I was keen to devise a plan and get working on the solution and to get quickly into a discussion about the treatment and beyond, but Doctor Nash was more cautious. He told me that many treatments were available and briefly outlined them for me but suggested that we await the results of the tests before we do anything else and on reflection, that seemed like a pretty sensible approach.

I thanked him for his time and walked from the examination room like a Texan cowboy who'd lost his horse, back to where Carol was waiting. At some time in the future I might look back on that moment as a time when the bottom fell out of my world, but right then I felt like the world was about to fall out of my bottom.

As we headed for home, Carol enquired about the ultrasound and I described the highlights (and the lowlights) to her. I said that the doctor would call me in a few days to let me have the results. It was clear to me now that the test was by way of confirmation of what the doctor and I both knew: **I had cancer**. - It's not a word that I had given much consideration to, nor did I feel that the full ramifications of it applied to me. Cancer was that awful thing that other unfortunate people get. What I had was some sort of nuisance factor we simply had to deal with. I didn't believe that it was a useful word to describe my condition and at that time I didn't feel that what was going on in my body was particularly serious. In that certainty I chose not to discuss it with Carol as we drove home. I knew her fear of cancer, having lost her sister to the disease at the early age of 25. I knew that she would see my condition in a far worse light than was the case. However, the main reason for not telling her there and then was that I would be working away from home for the rest of the week and didn't want to create any unnecessary anxiety in her mind whilst I was away. The next morning I headed off to Alabama.

# 4
# Making Choices

I didn't learn about the various treatments for prostate cancer and their side effects in any great detail until a few weeks after my diagnosis, but I'm visiting the subject now to help the reader become more informed than I chose to be. Obviously, when making decisions on which treatment may be most suitable, it is vital to do some proper research, which is exactly what I did some time later.[2]

When I read that "Cancer of the prostate has been described as a disease that men die *with* rather than *from*", I was reassured that my original feelings were correct and that this wasn't so serious. I also noted that approximately 42% of all men will develop cancer cells in the prostate during their lifetime but only about 3% of them will die of the disease. For many years people, including me, have placed prostate cancer in a category of being 'easily curable'. However, I realise now that we shouldn't be so dismissive of the seriousness of this disease. As the 35,000 deaths each year in the US indicate, prostate cancer is potentially lethal. It is one of the biggest killer cancers in men, second only to lung cancer. The most compelling point from my research, and one which resounded with me, is that cancer is an extremely fierce enemy requiring aggressive action. Usually, small measures don't eliminate it; they merely

---

[2] Sources of information used in this chapter come from the book – "His Prostate and Me", by Desiree Lyon Howe, from the pamphlet "What You Need To Know About Cancer" issued by the National Institute of Health and from fact sheets issued by the urologists' office.

stave off the day when it has to be confronted.

Following the introduction and widespread use of PSA in the USA and other improved diagnostic methods, prostate cancer can now frequently be identified at an early stage of development. This was quite a dilemma for me and for most other sufferers. Given that cancer is such a fierce disease, should I continue to live a normal life, leaving any treatment until the cancer became more serious, or should I take a major step straight away with the intention of eliminating the problem, hopefully for good? I started to realise that the choice is further complicated by the side effects of each of the treatment options. I have listed the various treatments here, in an order, which, in my personal view, ranges from the least to the most intrusive, and to a certain extent, the least to most effective. As you will see, in trying to make this choice you don't get 'owt for nowt'.

## 1. Watchful Waiting

As cancer of the prostate is reputed to be a slow-growth cancer, some men choose to monitor its growth, having PSA tests every six months or so and watching for the changes in their levels. My PSA was very low and many men with such a PSA are likely to opt for 'watchful waiting'. The theory is that it will be a long time before any treatment becomes necessary. Older men particularly favour this approach where there is a life expectancy of less than ten years.

The downside of 'watchful waiting' is that, since the cancer can be more aggressive or widespread than it may appear through PSA results alone, the sufferer may end up forfeiting his chance to be cured. Although some men are content to live with this uncertainty, like most other men, I was unwilling to put up with the worry that the cancer would be quietly growing and potentially escaping from the prostate, causing me to miss the 'window of opportunity.'

## 2. Hormone Therapy

Hormone therapy is a systemic approach used to control prostate cancer. The good news is that is almost always successful in reducing PSA for periods of six months to ten years or more. The bad news is that once the PSA starts to rise again, an alternative therapy will need to be used. Therefore, it is not a curative treatment and only works for a period of time, which varies between patients. Although the therapy is not realistically a front-line approach for prostate cancer, it is sometimes used as a pre or post treatment, in conjunction with other methods. It is also used as a stopgap for older men or those who cannot immediately undergo other treatments. The therapy works by shutting down the production of the male hormone testosterone, that 'feeds' the cancer.

The patient will almost always lose his libido (sex drive) for the duration of the treatment. In addition, he can expect to experience hot flushes, fatigue, breast enlargement, tenderness of the nipples, muscle loss and osteoporosis.

The alternative to chemical castration is the surgical removal of the testes or **orchidectomy** to give it its correct medical name. It is the quickest and most certain method of ridding the body of testosterone, thereby depriving the cancer cells of male hormones. The testosterone from the testes plummets within hours of the surgery and disappears permanently, along with any chance of normal sexual function. Although this is certainly an effective approach there is no chance of reversing the procedure. The obvious downside is its finality and the subsequent psychological effects of castration. For this reason, and the thought of having my balls cut off, I quickly dismissed this as forming any part of my pending treatment.

Whether a surgical or a chemical option is used in the process, it produces drastic responses. The PSA decreases and the tumour and any affected lymph nodes shrink.

I found the hormone treatment particularly interesting and wondered whether this might be a good approach for me, together with watchful waiting, allowing me to lead a near-normal life for a few years longer, before more drastic measures were needed.

### 3. Chemotherapy

Chemotherapy involves the use of toxic compounds to kill cancer cells. This has not been a particularly effective treatment for prostate cancer in the past, but is sometimes used in palliative care to relieve a patient's symptoms and improve his quality of life. It usually improves his overall health as well as minimising the intensity and duration of his pain. As chemotherapy is a palliative[3] treatment and still largely in a developmental stage, I haven't included any further detail here, although many books are available on the topic.

## 4. Cryotherapy

Freezing the prostate is a relatively easy, minimally invasive treatment option. Probes circulating liquid nitrogen are inserted into the prostate. The freezing process is monitored using ultrasound. The complete eradication of the tumour might require freezing the entire prostate, which could damage the urethra or the rectum. Very few cryotherapy treatments are performed, as the cancer is rarely completely eradicated and the side effects, such as erectile dysfunction[4] appear to be substantial.

## 5. Radiation

I was particularly interested to learn that early prostate cancer can be successfully treated with radiation therapy. Radiation destroys cancer cells by altering their capacity to reproduce or by inciting apoptosis, which is a self-destruction process causing cell death.

There are two main types of radiotherapy. One form is external beam radiation where the patient receives 35 to 40 high energy x-rays over a period of seven or eight weeks. The second form which is becoming more common is known as brachytherapy or seed therapy, as it involves the permanent implantation of minute radioactive "seeds" directly into the prostate

---

[3] Palliative treatments don't cure the underlying disease, but are used to treat the symptoms and improve the quality of life for a patient.
[4] The inability to get or maintain and erection

using ultrasound guidance.

Radiation, as a primary treatment, tends to be favoured for older men, because radiation may cure or slow the growth of their cancer and increase life expectancy to the point that they can live a substantial number of years free from symptoms and unaffected by the disease. Radiation therapy is not always curative, particularly with aggressive or widespread cancer, or if it has spread into the pelvis. However, it is a good option for patients like me who want to avoid the more invasive treatment of surgery.

Apart from mild incontinence and impotence problems, the patient may experience a variety of other symptoms: fatigue, diarrhoea, rectal pain and increased frequency in bowel activity, urinary urgency, irritated intestines or bladder irritation. Usually, these symptoms are only experienced for a few weeks after completion of the therapy but they vary in severity from patient to patient.

Problems with erectile dysfunction are initially less common with radiation than with surgery, although they are still frequent but may be delayed for up to 18 months because the cell damage occurs over a period whereas, with surgery, the problem is immediate. Radiation affects a man's erection by damaging the arteries and reducing blood flow to the penis. Depending on the nature of the damage, some men can regain potency over a period of time.

## 6. Radical Prostatectomy

A radical prostatectomy is one of the most difficult surgeries to perform; period. Although this is a fairly common procedure, it shouldn't be considered routine. The process involves cutting into the areas around the bladder and bowel and, if it isn't carried out correctly, can have significant side effects for many years. Therefore, the patient should try to do everything possible in advance to ensure the process is satisfactory. This includes choosing an excellent surgeon, (which may be easier said than done outside of the US), improving one's overall health and carefully following the doctor's orders

Most importantly, the procedure shouldn't be undertaken until at least six weeks after any biopsy, as the inflammation and punctures in the wall of the rectum caused by the procedure need time to heal. The inflammation causes the prostate to adhere to the rectum. If surgery were performed before the inflammation heals, the surgeon might have difficulty separating the two organs. This further complicates an already complicated surgery and could mean that the surgeon might not be able to remove all the cancer. It is also advisable to donate blood prior to the operation to be used in the event of blood loss during the surgery. The patient should take iron supplements and refrain from using blood-thinning medication before the donation takes place.

At one time, surgeons weren't aware that the tiny nerves necessary for achieving an erection were lying along both sides of the prostate, so they inadvertently cut them during the prostatectomy, thus leaving the man impotent. Now, by using nerve-sparing surgery, men are not automatically impotent after surgery.

Despite the surgeon's efforts to spare these nerves, damage can occur. Since the nerves control blood flow to the penis, the damage causes erection problems in 50-80 percent of patients who have a radical prostatectomy. The potency effect of this surgery is related to the man's age, the extent of the nerve sparing that is possible and the skill of the surgeon, or a combination of all of these factors. Most often, men under 60 years old, who have strong erections before surgery, are usually the ones who recover fully functional erections, particularly with the additional assistance of Viagra. However, regardless of their potency, they will still be able to have an orgasm. The only difference is that there won't be any sperm, and it will be a dry orgasm.

Unfortunately, nerve-sparing surgery cannot be performed on all men. As these tiny neurovascular bundles adhere to the surface of the prostate gland, if cancer is near or on the nerves already, it is unlikely that the nerve bundles can be spared and they will be removed, resulting in complete impotency.

Many men choose to have a radical surgery as their best hope of eliminating the cancer. Where cancer is confined to the prostate or has even penetrated into the wall or capsule it is usually cured by this method. If all of the cancer is removed, no further treatment is needed.

The most common surgical complications of the radical prostatectomy are excess bleeding and injuries to the rectum. Although only less than one percent of patients die during the surgery it remains a more difficult, invasive treatment than radiation.

---

For completeness, it should be understood that there is another situation, which I have not specifically included here. That is where the cancer has gone beyond the prostate, making it less treatable or, indeed, untreatable. However, even then the urologist will want to provide palliative care to do whatever can be done in slowing the inevitable outcome and making the patient more comfortable.

Although I have included quite a lot of detail here and in other chapters, the whole area of treatments and their side effects are complex far beyond my truncated explanation. However, armed with even this overview, it is clear that with such a wide choice of treatments available, varying in effectiveness and with a diverse number of side effects associated with each, this is not a straightforward choice. To complicate matters even further, occasions can arise where two or more treatments will be necessary to tackle the problem. It is therefore essential to fully understand what might suit each individual case. This needs to be done in close consultation with the urologist, although even he or she will have their own preferred treatments. As I said earlier, when I was facing this choice, I had much less understanding of the various treatments than I have included here, although, as will become clear later, a more detailed understanding wouldn't have assisted me in the decision.

# 5
## 'What's up Doc'?

I arrived on the early flight into Huntsville Alabama and picked up a hire car to head off for the chemical site in Decatur. I had slept well the night before and the news of the likelihood of cancer hadn't particularly disturbed me. My focus was on completing the second leg of a two-week study at site and as the team had had to work without me for a while, I needed to get things back on track and make sure we completed our objective before the end of the week. We made good progress during the day and after dinner that evening I went to my hotel room and typed up some notes before my bed started beckoning me. I decided to use the bathroom one last time, before turning in, and to my horror; I noticed that the water in the toilet bowl was taking on a distinct appearance of raspberry juice. The doctor had warned me that traces of blood could be present in the urine for a few days but I had not expected it to be quite so dramatic. This wasn't a trace; it looked more like an armful to me. I was frightened: I was a long way from home, from my doctor, and I felt completely alone. Through the night I kept monitoring things but it didn't seem to improve. I started to wonder whether the pressurisation of the airplane so soon after the biopsy, might have caused damage to my bladder. It hadn't occurred to me to check with the doctor about any concerns linked with flying before I left his surgery and now it was too late. I resolved that if it didn't calm down early in the morning, I would contact the nearest hospital. Soon after breakfast however, the bleeding stopped and I began to feel a little happier about things. Its funny how something that is apparently so serious, can become a distant thought, but that's how it was. By mid morning I had completely forgotten about it.

I made a phone call to Carol during the morning, to see how she was and to catch up with the news. I didn't mention the bleeding because I knew she would worry, and I was fine now. During the call she mentioned that the doctor's office had called and they wanted me to ring him sometime during the day. Given that he had tried to contact me so soon after the test, I was fairly sure that I knew what the news was going to be but my voice conveyed no concern to Carol regarding the message. I was trying to keep things on an even keel until I got back home. However, as I learned from her some days later, at this stage, she was already starting to think that it was bad news, but she hadn't worked out exactly how bad it might be.

After we ended our call, I rang the doctor's office but unfortunately, he was busy attending to another patient and was unable to come to the phone straight away. I left the telephone numbers of the location where I could be contacted, hoping that he would ring back soon. Crazy though it may seem now, for a variety of reasons all through Wednesday and Thursday we kept missing each other's calls. By Friday the work in Alabama was complete and I headed for the airport just before lunch. After checking in for my flight I decided to make a concerted effort to contact the doctor, before take-off. I had been steeling myself for the difficult task of breaking the grim news to Carol and, if cancer was confirmed, I needed to be armed with as much information as possible in order that I could answer all her inevitable questions. I knew it would be extremely difficult to console her but at least I wanted to be equipped with good information about the next steps although this was one weekend that I was really not looking forward to.

In my rush to get to the airport, I discovered I had mislaid the doctor's telephone number and decided to call Carol to get it. That call turned out to be one of the most painful moments of my life. Unbeknown to me, the doctor, frustrated at not being able to make contact with me during the week, had finally rung Carol as his office was about to close and he didn't want to leave us guessing over the weekend. He (wrongly) assumed that I had discussed his concerns from the biopsy with her and he proceeded to tell her the results of the test.

As soon as I said "hello" I knew something was wrong. I could hear Carol choking back the tears. There was a brief pause before she blurted out the words that she didn't want to say and I didn't want to hear. Through the tears and gasps for breath, I managed to make out her ominous message. "Doctor Nash has just rung me. I don't know how I can tell you …. Oh my God! You, you…..you've got cancer." At that point her controlled tears now turned into unrestrained sobbing. In an effort to calm and reassure her, I said, "I know that, I have known all week." Well of course, that didn't make things better; in fact it made things a whole lot worse. Clearly she was having such a difficult time, struggling with the news and with the thought of having to break it to me. My attempt at reassurance had just confirmed that I knew all along and had kept it from her. Apart from being distraught, she now felt betrayed as well. Any reaction I may have had to learning the reality of my situation was lost in the moment, out of a desire to protect her from this awful truth and to hold her close, to be strong for her and to stem her tears. However, I was hundreds of miles and three long hours travelling time away and that was going to have to wait. As we ended our call, I assured her that things would be OK. I asked her to hold things together until I got home, but that was cold comfort for her and empty sentiment from me. This was a life changing, and potentially life threatening, moment: things would never be quite the same from now on and I'd wanted to be with her to break the news myself. It was a task I'd dreaded and now the burden of telling her had been lifted. However, this didn't comfort me in any way. I didn't feel relieved, I only felt that I'd let her down badly and home seemed so far away. The next three hours seemed to last forever.

I picked up the phone once more and rang the doctor's office. Doctor Nash had already left for the weekend but his nurse informed me that he had left instructions for me to have a CT scan (or Cat scan as it's sometimes called) in order to determine how extensive the cancer was. As she spoke, I was thinking that trying to arrange a CT scan would be a lengthy process and enquired when it was likely to take place. She seemed a little surprised by my question and replied with equal surprise, "Well, next week, of course." I was taken aback. Up until now, the investigation of my prostate had been moving along at a steady pace. I was now about to learn exactly how efficient the medical system in the US is. I couldn't help reflecting on the fact that arranging a CT scan through the National Health Service would have taken weeks or months. In the US, it appeared, it was pretty well 'on demand'. Sure enough, before the following week was out I had the first of my many CT scans and booked an appointment with Doctor Nash on the following Tuesday to discuss the results.

The first day of November saw me back at the doctor's office. Carol was with me and we were both keen to learn the extent of the cancer and a lot more besides. We had dozens of questions and were hoping that Carol would be able to see the doctor with me; so that we could make sure we had the information clear in our minds. I was called into the office and Carol remained in the waiting room for now. The nurse weighed me and asked me to give a sample of urine, then showed me to a small examination room. As I sat waiting for the doctor, I looked at the various charts on the wall. They were useful for my further education, showing, amongst other things, the position of the prostate. At least I was getting to know a bit more about the workings of this body that I'd taken so much for granted over the last 50 odd years.

As I studied the charts the door opened but the person who entered the room was not Doctor Nash as I had expected, but a man who introduced himself as Doctor Freidman. He was in his late thirties I guessed and a Texan through and through. He explained that he was a senior consultant urologist and that Doctor Nash had suggested that he should pick up my case. He said that Doctor Nash had told him "you're a good guy and can handle the news head-on." He was right. I prefer it that way and don't like spending time beating around the bush. Well Doctor Freidman certainly was not one for beating around the bush either. He picked up my test results and said without any hesitation, "Well, man, you've got a hell of a lot of cancer up there." This was his way of telling me that I had advanced prostate cancer.

This straight talking was OK by me but I was glad that Carol was not there to hear it. I felt sure he was a good doctor but thought he could benefit from a course in bedside manners. He obviously wasn't big on words so he made sure that every one that tumbled from his lips made maximum impact. His straight talking was to be an ongoing feature of our relationship and I welcomed it, but he never ceased to surprise me in the way that he confronted the issues.

In true urologist fashion he asked me to drop my trousers and pants so that he could carry out a digital rectal examination. Well, there was no confusion in my mind. Not this time. I knew exactly what was in store and meekly lowered myself over the end of the examination couch while his inquisitive digit plunged its way towards my prostate. Freidman was clearly 'hands-on'. His examination technique was thorough: so thorough in fact that I thought it would never end. Every now and again he would let out a soft 'Hmm" to himself and then move his 'digit' to another position. Eventually he was finished and he confirmed that it was certainly an unusual shape.

"Not what I would expect from someone with a PSA of less than four!" he exclaimed. He pondered for a few more seconds and then, reaching for the door handle, announced that this was so unusual that he was going to invite a colleague to take a look. I wouldn't have minded if he really meant that he would look but I knew this was a euphemistic phrase for another DRE.

As I stood there waiting with my trousers around my ankles, I was starting to wonder just what it was about my prostate that caused a whole team of urologists to plunder my rectum with their rubber-gloved fingers. My mind wandered and, in order to pass the time and not dwell on this invasion of my anatomy by the whole medical practice, I tried to think up a collective noun for a group of urologists. I finally decided on handful: 'A handful of urologists'. I was hoping that I wasn't too far off the mark. This colleague was going to be the fourth to carry out a DRE and I knew my rectum would struggle to cope with more than a handful.

By the time his colleague arrived, I'd stopped considering the benefits of having doctors with small hands for this type of examination. I think that only holds true for the first one. After that, it starts to matter less. All I wanted now was for the whole experience to be over and I was hoping that if he had any other colleagues that might find my prostate interesting, they would be out of the office, on holiday, off sick or anywhere but here. Not that a DRE is particularly painful, but neither is it my idea of a fun day out.

His colleague was pulling on his rubber gloves as he

entered the room. He flashed me a casual smile, which I took as my signal and bent across the end of the couch again. As I did so, he took his turn at examining my prostate. He muttered words of agreement to Freidman as he left the room and I realised that he had carried out the DRE without even speaking a word in my direction. I couldn't help thinking that a polite, "excuse me" or "thank you" wouldn't have gone amiss. As I dressed myself and sat down, very carefully, the nurse showed Carol into the room for our discussion with Freidman.

Since men generally are not inclined to communicate their questions or elaborate on more than their basic symptoms to doctors, I found having Carol present, particularly helpful. Discussions of any detail can be quite bewildering; when you have just been diagnosed as having prostate cancer (or any cancer for that matter) making it difficult to remember much of the conversation with the doctor after the visit. It is a good idea to take notes and to have some pertinent questions prepared beforehand. I have included a sample of frequently asked questions in Appendix A which may help during any such discussion.

For Carol and me, the first question we faced after diagnosis was, "What do we do next?" I intentionally say "we" because in my experience, both personal and through talking with other prostate cancer survivors, prostate cancer is a condition, which affects the partner, almost as much as the patient. I believe that it was essential to involve Carol at this early stage of the process; otherwise she would be playing catch-up, which might cause misunderstanding and resentment later.

## Brian Turner

In most situations, in order to make the right decision, an understanding of the treatment options is essential. There is an enormous benefit in talking them through with the urologist and, if possible, with prostate cancer survivors. At my previous meeting with Doctor Nash he had made me aware of different treatment options and I had carried out a bit of research, (as outlined in chapter four), in readiness for this discussion. In my mind I'd decided to go for the hormone therapy (although, I had immediately dismissed any idea of an orchidectomy: the mere thought bringing tears to my eyes) and enjoy my life for a few more years without too much disruption. I was convinced that if that didn't do the trick, I could always go for a more intrusive treatment at some time in the future. That way, I could put off the evil day when I might have to give up my potency. (I'd obviously missed the fact that hormonal therapy reduces testosterone). After all, at fifty-one I was still in my prime.

As it turned out, we spent no time discussing the various treatment options. This was to be one of those 'Oh Fuck!' moments in life, which sometimes present themselves but you wish you didn't have to face up to. Doctor Freidman's message was clear and unequivocal: based on my Gleason reading of 4+4 from the biopsy and the feel of my prostate, there was only one option: Radical surgery. I had read a bit about the Gleason scale and proud of my recently acquired knowledge said, "Well, four is pretty good, isn't it?" to which Freidman shook his head and replied that it would make things more complicated. He said that he would have preferred it to be 3+3 and subsequently, as the organ was so full of cancer, there would be no chance of nerve sparing surgery. This was to be the "Full Monty".

As I sat pondering the news and what it all meant, he came out with another observation, in his own inimitable style. "How are your erections?" he enquired. I told him with some pride that they were fine thank you. His retort was another classic, no-nonsense statement. "Well, after the operation you won't be able to get an erection." I thought bloody hell! This is obviously not good news week, but his point didn't escape me. Although losing the ability to have an erection was not a situation I relished, it was a small price to pay given that the alternative was so awful and eventually, much more final.

With the news still ringing in our ears, we left the doctor's office and drove off towards home. We were both silent for a while: I was still trying to work out the significance of the Gleason indicator of 4+4. I obviously hadn't taken a great deal of care in my reading but recalled something about the scale being in two parts and the score then being averaged for the final, single-digit reading. As the maximum on the scale is ten, I was still of the impression that four was pretty good in the scheme of things and couldn't understand why the doctor didn't appear to echo my sentiment. I made a mental note to do a bit more research on the subject.

Lost in my own thoughts of Gleason, I was completely unaware of what was going on in Carol's mind, but she broke the silence and enquired in a matter-of-fact kind of way, "Well, what do you think?" It was a fairly general question but I knew for sure she wasn't referring to the weather or what plans we may have for the rest of the day. I knew she would be struggling with the news but I told her that this was so much easier than I'd expected, to which she gave me a really quizzical look. Trying to clarify things for her, I said, "Well, deciding on the treatment was a bit like opening my wardrobe and finding only one pair of trousers hanging there. There's absolutely no point in spending any time wondering what you're going to do when there is only one choice."

When we arrived home, the nurse rang to confirm the date of my operation. It was to be on 12th December, with a pre-op appointment a week earlier. I checked the calendar – it was only 6 weeks away.

# 6
## Gleason Revealed

I decided that I needed to know a lot more about the cancer that was causing the problem and, for that matter, where my prostate actually was and what it did for a living, so over the next few weeks, I started surfing the web to get myself better informed. I was also keen to get more reliable information about the grading method that Doctor Gleason had come up with and for which I was still trying to get clear in my mind.

*"Normally, body cells grow and divide to form new cells in an orderly way. After they have performed their function for a while, they die and other cells take their place. This is the usual way that a healthy body is sustained. However, sometimes the cells don't die but keep dividing and creating more cells that the body doesn't need. This eventually causes a build up of tissue called a tumour. These tumours can be benign or malignant.*

*"Benign tumours are not cancer. If necessary, they can usually be removed and even if they are not, will not spread to other parts of the body and they pose no threat to life. On the other hand, malignant tumours* **are** *cancer and they contain abnormal cells, which grow out of control and are without order – and they don't die. These malignant cells can break away from the main tumour and enter the bloodstream and lymphatic system. This spread of cancer is known as metastasis.*

*"The medical profession does not yet understand the causes of prostate cancer, although studies have appeared to highlight risk factors associated with the disease.*

- ***Age.** Prostate cancer is mainly found in men over the age of 55, although the average age of a patient at the time of diagnosis is 70.*
- ***History.** A man is at higher risk from prostate cancer if his father or a male sibling has had the disease.*
- ***Race.** The disease is much more common in African American men than in white men, although it is least common in Asians.*
- ***Diet.** There is evidence to suggest that a diet that is high in animal fat may increase the risk of prostate cancer, while a diet high in fruit and vegetable content may decrease the risk. Studies are ongoing to determine whether certain dietary supplements would reduce the occurrence.*
- ***Other.** Studies have suggested having a vasectomy may increase the risk of prostate cancer. In addition, obesity, lack of exercise, smoking, radiation exposure and sexually transmitted viruses have all been cited as risk factors, although, at this time there is little evidence to support these factors as contributing to the overall risk.*

"The prostate is a gland in the male reproductive system and is about the size and shape of a walnut. It is located in front of the rectum, just below the bladder and it surrounds the urethra. The urethra is the organ that carries urine from the bladder out through the penis.

## Please Leave The Seat Up

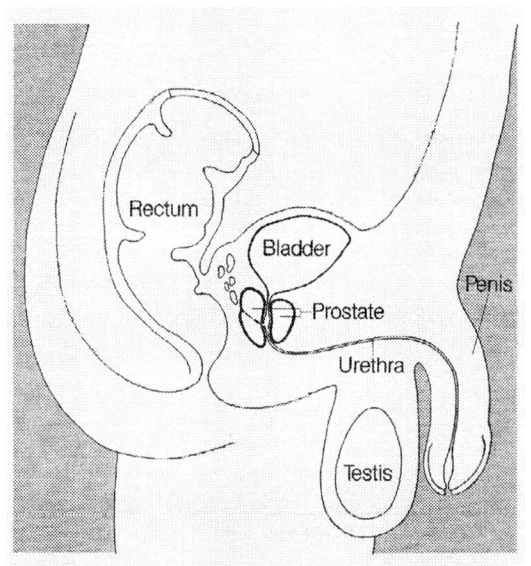

This picture shows the prostate and nearby organs.

*"The prostate is made up of thousands of tiny fluid-producing glands. More specifically, it is an exocrine gland: so-called because it secretes through ducts to the outside of the body. (Sweat glands are another example of an exocrine gland.) The fluid produced by the prostate forms part of semen, the fluid that carries sperm during orgasm. This fluid is stored with sperm in the seminal vesicles and during male sexual climaxes; muscular contractions cause the prostate to secrete this fluid into the urethra, where it is expelled from the body through the penis.*

*"In addition, the prostate also has a major role in controlling the flow of urine. The prostate wraps itself*

*around the upper part of the urethra as it passes from the bladder to the penis. The muscular fibres in the prostate contract to stop the flow of urine at times between normal urination.*

*"In order to work correctly, the prostate needs male hormones (androgens). Male hormones are responsible for male sex characteristics. The main male hormone is testosterone, which is made mostly in the testicles, although some of the male hormones are produced by the adrenal glands."*[5]

This all sounded somewhat clinical for me, but even with my limited grasp of medical terminology, I now realised that the prostate was essential for having sex and peeing. As I was about to lose control over both of these, it certainly helped to focus my mind.

Doctor Freidman had informed me that all six of my biopsy samples were positive and my Gleason score was noted in the laboratory report as 4+4. As you will recall, I'd read a bit about Gleason and by my reckoning, 4+4 was a Gleason reading of 4, which on a scale of 1 to 10 didn't seem all that bad. However, Freidman had also told me that this was a very important number and he was concerned that the reading was at 4+4 rather than 3+3 so I was really keen to understand why. As part of my research, I obtained a fact sheet from the urologist's office, which revealed the nature of my misunderstanding. I have used extracts from the document to help me with the explanation, rather than continue

---
[5] Extract from "What You Need to Know about Prostate Cancer" a pamphlet issued by the National Institute of Health.

to compound my previous error, thereby leaving the reader as ill-informed as I obviously was.

*"The scores are given as the pathology test results from a grading system developed by Doctor Donald Gleason[6]. It's used to measure the aggressiveness of the tumour by looking at glandular patterns under a microscope. Normal glands are uniform in appearance with a layer of two cells. The cancerous glands have a single layer of cells and become more and more irregular and disorganised until they are a mishmash of diseased looking cells. When pathologists study the different biopsy samples, they look to determine differing patterns in the various parts of the prostate. Until Dr. Gleason described five specific categories or "grades" of such tumour patterns, classifying the cancer was more difficult.*

*"Grade 1 glands are well organized and differentiated in appearance and look almost like benign tissue. This grade is very rare, since the cells in most tumours have progressed beyond this level before they can be detected by the DRE or PSA. Grade 5 glands are so poorly organized that they are uniform sheets of cells with no glandular organisation. A grade 5 is quite rare because the tumour is usually diagnosed before it reaches this level. As one might expect, a Gleason grade of three is the one most commonly found, because it is mature enough to be detected through DRE and PSA tests, but not so mature that the treatment options are limited. Interestingly, the higher the Gleason*

---
[6] Doctor Gleason is the reference pathologist for the Veterans Cooperative Group.

*grade the less PSA the cells generate, which would suggest that when a patient is nearing the top end of the Gleason scale, his PSA may be relatively low.*

*"To determine the Gleason score, the pathologist finds the tumour with the highest volume and allocates it a grade between 1 and 5. Then the tumour with the second highest volume is determined and given a score of 1 to 5. The Gleason score is the sum of the two grades, (*and not the average, as I'd previously imagined). *Therefore, Gleason scores can range from two (1+1) to ten (5+5). The Gleason score is extremely important since it indicates how aggressive the tumour might be. The most common is six (3+3). There are many sevens (3+4 or 4+3). Sevens are significantly more aggressive than the sixes and the 4+3's are more aggressive than the 3+4's. The differences between the scores are very significant. For example, a Gleason-6 tumour might be doubling every two to four years, while a Gleason-8 tumour might take two to four months and a Gleason-10 just two to four weeks."*

I was beginning to understand why, with a Gleason score of 8, the doctor was concerned about the aggressiveness of my own particular tumour. It was in both lobes and had penetrated into the capsule on both sides of the prostate and potentially had already "gotten out of the box" as Freidman had put it. This was definitely not the straightforward case I'd originally thought, although the true significance of the situation wouldn't fully register with me until I was on the operating trolley.

Again, I am quoting directly from the urologists' fact sheet: *"Another very important, routine determination is the 'Stage' of the cancer. This is an assessment of the physical extent of the cancer defined by clinical results using the DRE, transrectal ultrasound (TRUS), biopsy, bone scans, CT scans, etc. Staging is beneficial in determining the appropriate treatment for a specific case, because knowing the location and extent of the tumour allows the physicians to be more precise in their treatment recommendations.*

*"The international TNM staging system is the most common staging system used. The 'T' indicates the primary Tumour in the prostate. The 'N' ranking characterises the extent of lymph Node involvement, if any, and the 'M' specifies whether a cancer has Metastasized (passed to another part of the body) beyond the lymph nodes.*

*"Combining these three rankings gives a quick summary of the tumour and a more understandable way to determine the best therapy for the patient. The T-N-M rankings have subsets of numbers and letters, which are even more definitive, and complicated. The doctor will clearly suggest a different course of treatment for a patient with a T3-N2-MO ranking than will be the case for someone with a T2-NO-MO. The ranking table is set out in Appendix B as an indication of how this works.*

At the preliminary stage, my rating was T3-NX-M1a, but as I hadn't researched the staging process, this meant nothing to me at that time. However, when

*Brian Turner*

I received the pathology reading some months later it helped paint a much clearer picture for me.

# 7
# Sharing the News

Having found out where my prostate lay, Carol made sure I also knew where my priorities lay. One of the first things she said following my diagnosis was that the treatment must take first place and work will have to come second for a change. As she looked me in the eye, I knew that, on this occasion, there was to be no compromise. Not that one was needed as far as I was concerned. I was now firmly aware of what was required and although work had always come first with me, often at the expense of important personal matters, this was different. For the first time in my career I was ready, nay determined, that my work had to be lower down my priority order. I have always had a 'can do' attitude, avoiding trying to find obstacles where none exists. This has allowed me to approach life in a positive and optimistic way, rather than always assuming the worst. Right from the start, I'd taken the view that whatever was necessary to be done to eradicate the cancer, should be done without compromise. However, my approach was to avoid looking too far forward to all the complications that could arise with the surgery and beyond. I was determined not to be panicked into worrying about how bad things could get, preferring to take it one step at a time. Where things stood at present, I had cancer in my prostate and I was going to have it surgically removed. I had no reason to concern myself with the problems, which may or may not arise later. After all, I was generally in good health and took the view that the operation would get the cancer beaten once and for all.

Obviously, prostate cancer isn't good news but I didn't think that having it surgically removed was any big deal. After all, it's merely an operation to remove an unwanted part of the body. I thought of it as being similar to when I had my appendix removed when I was 14 years old. I was soon back up and about, playing with my toys. Mind you, I did string it out a bit longer than was strictly necessary as it meant I could stay off school for a while. But now I was a mature adult with a keen sense of responsibility and a real enthusiasm for my work. Getting this operation done and out of the way was going to be easy by comparison. I was expecting to have the surgery mid December, and then recover during the Christmas break, returning to work early in the New Year. As most people I was working with were busy with their own holiday arrangements during the period, it was a great opportunity to use the time effectively, rather than screw up my busy work schedule. How wrong could I have been!

As I wasn't treating this as a big deal, I was reticent about sharing the news more widely. Not out of any embarrassment or modesty, (as Carol is quick to remind me, modesty is not my strong point) but I suppose in those early days after the diagnosis, I believed there was no need to make a fuss. I had obviously had experience of friends and family with cancer, but somehow felt that this was different. In my mind, this wasn't real cancer, it was only *prostate cancer* which many men experience in their life, and therefore, getting through it was hardly worth a mention. I really only needed to tell those people where it may impact on other arrangements: In short, probably this would be only a handful of people. Nor did it occur to me that people would have any interest or feel the need to share the news with other friends and colleagues. I could never have imagined that I might become the centre of interest of so many people. In the first few weeks I only mentioned it to a few: a couple of work colleagues and my sister, who then took on the responsibility of briefing the wider family. However, as time went on, I realised that I would need to share the news more widely, but the problem was that most of those I needed to share it with were a whole continent away and this is not the type of news to try and relay over the telephone.

My biggest priority was to advise my boss, Kevin, who was based in London. An important business meeting was coming up in the UK, which needed my input. I could have tackled it on a telephone conference call, but we all felt it would be better handled face-to-face and I realised that it was the perfect opportunity to share the news with Kevin. As I boarded my flight for the meeting, I also saw this as the opportunity to brief a few of my friends and family face-to-face. However, over the next few days I was to find out that I'd been totally unprepared for their reactions.

I had learned fairly early on in the process (as if it were not already self-evident) that people generally have a real difficulty talking about cancer. In my view, it is largely because they are never quite sure what to say or how the sufferer may be feeling and dealing with it in their own mind. When the 'cancer patient' informs them that he or she has the disease, ether an uncomfortable silence follows, accompanied by the shuffling of feet, or the person looks genuinely shocked or surprised and appears to want to hug the patient in order to make them feel better. When words finally come, it is usually to say how sorry they are, as if they are somehow at fault. Clearly, what they mean is that they feel sorrow that you have the disease but it often sounds that, by some curious way, they have had some personal responsibility for you having been selected to endure cancer. Their next consideration is usually an offer to help in any way they can. Although this is always a genuine and heartfelt offer, people are never quite sure what it might entail.

In my experience, few people have a natural ease dealing with the news. This is only to be expected, as most people's experience of the dreaded 'C word' is surrounded by visions of a period of long and unpleasant suffering, before the patient finally drifts into a near comatose state, slipping away to a happy release. At least, they are the experiences which stick in one's mind. I believe that this is the mental picture most people have when they receive the news of cancer affecting a friend or loved one.

When people offer help on learning about one's cancer, they really mean it in the literal sense. They are keen to do whatever they can to help. They become almost as frustrated as the sufferer to learn that the only people who can deal with the major issue, the actual treatment of the cancer, are the experts in the medical profession: the doctors and nurses, the urologists, the radiologists and the whole entourage of specialists who the patient will become so dependent on over the months ahead. For the patients and their friends, help usually comes down to support, good wishes and prayer. But for most people this doesn't feel adequate. They want to *do* something and in reality, there is very little to physically *do*.

When I started to share my news with friends, I was able to understand this type of reaction better, having lost my own mother to cancer just prior to her 75th birthday two years previously. She died six short weeks after the diagnosis of cancer in her oesophagus and during that time, we all wanted to do something. Sure, we spent time with her, made her laugh and shared in her bouts of pain, we fed her and kept her comfortable; and we loved her. But she knew what we all knew - she was dying. She was strong for us all, right to the end, but we always felt that we wanted to do something. It was with this experience that I realised when people started to offer me their help that they couldn't know what the "doing" would involve. In reality, prayer, support and help are every bit as important as the treatment itself. A significant benefit is achieved and, by just being there, friends are indeed doing the things that are needed; plugging the gaps and taking over when the medical profession has done their bit, showing interest in the progress and treatment, and simply being supportive.

I found that breaking the news to people was much trickier than I'd anticipated. In my mind, this was merely information, but from other people's perspective, it was tragic and they gushed with sympathy, which I found embarrassing and unnecessary. At first, people's reactions were quite a shock to me and the reaction of my daughter, Sharon, a 30-year-old publican, was one that surprised me the most. She had always been so level-headed and robust and I felt she had the capacity to deal with almost anything that life could throw at her. I'd advised her that I would be in the UK for a week and would like to meet up with her. At first she was pleased to get an opportunity for a get together, even though she lived in Somerset and I was in London. As we started to work out the details, it was proving difficult to find a time when she could get away from work and as my week was full of work-related things in town and around Manchester, it looked like we were not going to pull it off. However, I was determined not to let the opportunity of telling her face-to-face pass us by, and started to suggest more drastic steps, which included my driving to Somerset and back one evening. She was clearly trying to spare me the ordeal and suggested that if we couldn't make it fit, we should agree to meet up the next time I was over.

By now I was getting panicky and insisted that we had to meet as I needed to tell her something important. We finally agreed on a plan and I thought that I would now be able to deliver the news unhindered. However, Sharon had obviously started to mull over all the things that could be so urgent that I had to tell her now – and in person - and came to the conclusion that this was going to be news she didn't want to hear. Within a few minutes, she had rung back and made an excuse as to why we couldn't meet as arranged and once again I was left wondering how I could make this work. As I sat and pondered our discussions, all the while getting more and more concerned as to whether we would get together, I struck on a master plan. As I knew she would be working that evening, I upped sticks and drove to Somerset. When I walked into the pub, she took one look at me and covered her ears, saying, "Don't tell me. Don't tell me." But it was too late and obviously I did tell her. When I reassured her that I was going to be fine, she calmed down and was happy to see me. We sat and chatted for a long time after the pub closed, catching up on lost time into the small hours, before I had to leave.

Later that week I was to learn even more about the consequences of sharing the news; it was brought home to me when I told Ian, a long-standing friend and work colleague. We had arranged to spend an afternoon with Ian, his wife Wendy and their two boys, Aaron and Aidan. Ian had just picked up a new car and was keen to show it off to me, so we went out for a 'test drive'. This was a good opportunity for me to tell him my news and it avoided us discussing it in front of the young boys. Ian and I had worked closely together on many projects and had a rough and macho approach to everything, bordering on arrogance. (Maybe I'm lying about the 'bordering' bit). I knew Ian would want to know my news, as we shared most things with each other, but I hadn't considered any reaction he may have other than to say something like 'tough luck, mate!' I was in the driving seat – so to speak – as we toured around the country lanes putting the new BMW through its paces.

During a break in the conversation, of which not

many occurred, I said casually, "I just wanted to let you know that I'm having an operation for prostate cancer in December," and added as an afterthought, "It's not a problem, but I need to have it done."

As a Sales Director, Ian is a man who speaks for a living and in all the years I have known him, I have never seen him short of words, even on many tricky occasions where I would have been struggling. As I concentrated on a sharp right-hand bend in the road, I was aware that Ian wasn't speaking and wondered if he was more concerned about my ability to take this bend than I was. After all, I had perfect control of the Beamer, which was singing like a bird as we clipped past the hedgerows. As we came out of the bend and I straightened the car up, I looked over to him, awaiting his next sarcastic comment on my driving skills, but nothing came. After a few more seconds I enquired if he was OK and he looked forlornly at me and said, "I'm stunned, mate! I don't know what to say – I just don't know what to say."

Oh shit! This was not the reaction I expected or wanted. I was feeling laid back about it and felt that Ian would have been much the same way. However, his reaction hit me like a stone and nearly brought me to tears. I realised then that if he, with our usual manly approach to things, could feel so shocked by the news, it was time for me to face up to the fact that telling people this information was going to be difficult. But difficult or not, I had to deal with it.

I met up with several other friends and relatives during my visit that week, and the reactions were generally the same. I finally acceded to their emotions and began to understand how much this was affecting them. I learned to deliver the message with more measure and assured people that I was OK about it. I found myself having to reassure everyone that I was going to be all right, and that they didn't need to be concerned. Of course they all offered to do anything they could, which was very kind. But I needed nothing except their support, which, in the end, proved to be the most valuable gift they could have given me.

You know what they say about the best-laid plans of mice and men? Since the unexpected reactions I'd had recently, I made a pact with myself that I wasn't going to tell people about my cancer over the phone unless it was absolutely necessary. I had arranged a meeting with Kevin for Wednesday and would tell him then. I would have liked the meeting to be sooner as I was a concerned that he may learn it from others before I got the opportunity to tell him myself, although it was unlikely, as he didn't know the few people who I'd already told. I was on my way back from Somerset on Tuesday afternoon and at about 3.00 p.m. I had a call on my mobile from a work colleague to advise me that Kevin was calling a meeting for 4.00 p.m. and asked if I could join the meeting by phone. I said I could and asked the purpose of the meeting. He told me it was a planning meeting to decide how to allocate the resources of our small team over the next six months and said calmly, "Speak to you at four," as he hung up.

I sat thinking for a few moments and decided that

I couldn't leave things like this. It would be an awful waste of everyone's time to discuss plans, when I knew that, at the very least, I would be absent from work for a month, which would blow the plan apart. I rang back into the office to discover that Kevin was in a meeting until 4.00, and I could see this all going badly wrong. The last thing I wanted was to make a grand announcement during the meeting, which deflected everyone from the business in hand. I left a message that Kevin must ring me urgently, **before** the meeting started. And so it was that at bang on the dot of four, and against my better judgment, I was sharing my news with Kevin over the phone. We quickly agreed to speak again later and I couldn't help thinking how ironic it was that I'd spent so much time, effort and company money on the trip to avoid such a situation, only to be thwarted by dint of this unscheduled meeting. As they say, timing is everything – but not in this case.

When I spoke with Kevin again, he was really magnificent. I was trying to warn him that I might be away from work for a month or so while I recover from the operation. We did the sympathy bit before we moved to more practical things and he was quick to tell me not to worry about work, but to concentrate on getting myself fit again saying, "Maybe it'll be a month but it will take as long as it takes and we will manage around it." Although he was preaching to the converted, I was glad that I had his wholehearted support. We spoke for quite a while on the phone that evening and even then, Kevin rang back twice more with some afterthoughts. The next morning he rang again and told me that he had spoken with Gill, the HR manager, overnight. They had been discussing a whole load of issues related to my situation, which I hadn't even thought of. Gill had offered to meet with Carol and me. She was keen to discuss how the company might help us through the many difficulties that may present themselves during my treatment We were pleased to have the opportunity and made an appointment to meet on the following Monday.

By the weekend, we were both washed out and decided to stay in the hotel, even though there were still plenty more people we hadn't seen. We invited my eldest sister, Betty, over for lunch and a chat. She is a good listener and we were all able to talk openly about the cancer; its affect on Carol and how we would deal with it. I didn't realise it then but Betty was going to play a key role over the next six months by taking responsibility for communicating with the family. I have seven siblings and she acted as the conduit for the flow of information between us all by giving updates of my progress to the others throughout my treatment. This helped cut down on the number of phone calls to and from the US, which at times were quite distressing and a real burden to Carol.

Our meeting with Gill the following Monday was extremely helpful and she was particularly good with Carol, offering her some real practical help, for which we were both grateful. Early on Tuesday morning we boarded the plane for home. It had been quite a week.

# 8
# Preparing for the Chop

After we had returned home from our trip to the UK, life moved on apace and I had a lot to do. The doctor had advised me to get in better shape before the operation, recommending that I start taking a whole range of vitamins including zinc, selenium, magnesium and calcium. He also advised me that he wanted me to have plenty of anti-oxidants to start fighting the free radical cancer. He told me that this was present in foods in the lycopene category. The list included tomatoes and tomato products, including pizza, pink grapefruit, watermelon, papaya and apricots In fact, it would appear he wanted me to concentrate on anything red because included in his list were cranberry juice and red wine. I liked that bit; at last I had found a doctor who prescribed alcohol as a medicine: Excellent. Unfortunately, he also wanted me to eat plenty of soy products, which is my least favourite food. Perhaps I could wash it down with a fine bottle of 1994 Chateau Neuf du Pape.

Most of all he wanted me to 'get fit' and increase my cardio-vascular rate. It occurred to me that he was telling me two years too late but, with such a limited time before the operation, I wasn't going to waste another second in putting this right. After nearly clearing the shelves of vitamins at the local pharmacy, I went to the wellness centre at the office and told the trainer that I needed a fitness programme in a hurry. Looking at his diary he suggested that we have a session on Thursday of next week. I told him that my needs were more immediate and so he reappraised his suggestion to the end of the week as an alternative.

"How about right now?" I said, taking him by surprise. He looked at me as I swung my sports bag off my shoulder and added, 'there's not a moment to waste – I'll go and get changed." And so it was that I started on a manic regime to undo all the damage those fifty odd years of abuse had done to my body. I wasn't expecting miracles but if I ever needed to work out, it was now.

As he grew to understand my urgent requirements, the trainer set out a plan of action for me. He was keen to slow me down, suggesting that if I went at it like I was suggesting, there would be no need for any operation as I would die of a heart attack long before then.

I had always considered that I had a 'fit for purpose' body. Unfortunately, the purpose it was fit for was sitting down (and then, only if I couldn't lie down instead) drinking lots of beer and eating good food in ample quantities. With great effort, I heaved my 258lbs of carefully honed masculinity onto the treadmill and started off. No running for me just yet. The equivalent of a casual stroll to the corner shop was about my limit, and even then, I needed a rest before the return journey. Every day I would jump - well eventually, in the beginning it was more like a lunge - on the machine in earnest, stepping up the pace a little every day. When I was back in the UK for a week, I paced the streets if I couldn't find a gym at the hotels I stayed in. Unfortunately, winter in the UK is somewhat colder than winter in Texas and as I went off on my early morning walks, I really had to step it out in order to prevent any of the metal bits that monkeys are purported to have – dropping off.

As I made progress with the keep fit, I felt that I could maximise the effort if I could incorporate additional exercise, so Carol and I set off for the cycle shop to get ourselves some glittering examples of the machine that Mr Raleigh had been so famous for in the UK. I was surprised just how much they had changed since I last sat on one, realizing that it must have been over thirty years. As we eyed this vast array of bikes the salesman, whom I suspect had a much grander title – *Vice President of Cycle Technology and Engineering*, or something similar, I wouldn't wonder – asked what we were looking for. "A bike," I stated clearly enough for every one to hear. He smiled and gave me a look, which told me that he thought I was a bit of a saddo who had wandered off the streets with no particular aim, except to muck up his day.

"What type of 'bike' did sir have in mind?" he asked sarcastically. Sir actually had absolutely no idea but sir wasn't about to admit it to the VP of CT&E, although I think he had already worked it out for himself. I simply moved further into the shop, trying to look nonchalant and knowledgeable. I grabbed the handlebars of the nearest bike on display and twisted them a couple of times, as if that were the normal method of testing a bike's roadworthiness.

"Is the cycle for your wife, sir?" he enquired. "Only you realise that is a lady's cycle." I wasn't going to be phased by this and casually mentioned that we actually wanted a bike each. However, by now any credibility I had was long gone, but I'm glad to report that the VP gave us a lot of help and information, allowing us to 'hit the street' with two gleaming 'bikes', although I was mildly amused when he told us that we only needed safety helmets if we were going to cycle in the parks. If we were planning to cycle on the highway, then Texas law didn't require them to be worn. It got me wondering exactly what it was that was lurking in the bushes of Texas parks that could make them so dangerous. Conversely, I deduced that if the same dangers weren't present on the road, maybe the tarmac was coated with foam rubber for a soft landing. Curious, eh? As we left the shop with our gleaming bikes, complete with safety headgear, he was muttering something about us being equipped to cycle up mountains, but it went way over my head.

---

After our return home from the UK, I continued to go to work as normal but each day got more complicated, as people tried to fix appointments to see me. They would suggest a date in early December and I would tell them that it was not available, then they would suggest "any day in December" and once again I would tell them I couldn't make it. Finally they would ask what dates were free in January and I would have to admit that I didn't know. Short of telling people why I couldn't make it, I had to keep things vague and tell them I would get back to them with some suggested dates in a week or so.

During that week, I attended the local blood bank. I had given blood many times before although this time it was different. I knew the recipient well, almost intimately you might say. This blood was for me. I had been advised that donating blood, which could be used during my operation if required, would reduce the possibility of an infection. That was good enough for me. I would have happily donated an armful for such a good cause.

Having spent more than an hour with Gill, the HR manager, before we left the UK, I was really surprised to see her in the Houston office on Wednesday of the following week, particularly as she hadn't mentioned that she was coming. It soon became apparent that she was there to see me. She told me that the leadership team had discussed my situation at length and had decided to grant me indefinite leave from close of work on Friday. I felt that it was an unnecessary offer as my operation was still a few weeks away but she insisted. In the end, it proved to be a blessing, as I didn't have to keep my work colleagues guessing about my schedule and it allowed me time to concentrate on my fitness. Carol was delighted when I told her.

As the operation drew nearer, we were both preparing for it in our own ways. Unbeknown to me, Carol kept sliding off to Barnes & Noble, the local bookshop, to read about prostate cancer in various books. She purchased one and read it in secret. However, it worried her so much that she hid it so that I didn't stumble across it accidentally. Finally, she couldn't bear to have the book in the house, so she took it back to the shop and got a refund[7] as she felt that I would be as equally worried by its content as she had been. What she hadn't realised was that my biggest worry was much more basic than that.

I'd had this feeling before. When I was a boy I would sometimes run an errand for a neighbour and earn myself a few coppers, only to find that it was two minutes to closing time at the sweetshop and to make matters worse, it wouldn't open again for two days, as tomorrow was Sunday. The frustration then was awful and it felt much the same now, only this particular sweetshop was not just about to close, but the whole sweet industry was going to be demolished overnight and my pennies (or my penis in this case) would be useless before I got the chance to pay another visit. I had managed to get my mind around impotency longer term but while I was fully functional, I couldn't stop thinking about it. Having been married for over twenty years, we had long passed the stage where sex was the only thing we thought about. We were much more comfortable with each other and our lovemaking was far less frequent than those heady days when we first met but we were content with the way things were. That was before I'd been put on notice that it was all going to come to an abrupt end on 12th December. Now, it was in my mind constantly. All this time, Carol was so distressed that it wasn't something I really wanted to bring up. Every day I felt that time and opportunity was slipping by and my

---
[7] We subsequently re-purchased the book, entitled 'His Prostate and Me' by Desiree Lyon Howe, after the operation and I found it immensely informative.

frustration was increasing. It started to feel like a loud screaming in my head. When we were out shopping, I would steer Carol to Victoria's Secret lingerie store and point out the pretty items of underwear in the window, but she didn't get my drift.

I thought that a break away from home would be useful. It would help to relax us both and create an atmosphere where I could 'spend my penny'. Carol agreed to a holiday but did nothing to advance the cause, like looking at glossy brochures or coming up with ideas of where to go. She didn't seem to be able to give time to thinking about it - and I couldn't stop thinking about it.

It was 3rd December and with time running out. I was due at the hospital at 9.00 a.m. for my pre-op checks. I was up early, as is my habit, so was working on my computer at around 6.00 a.m. As I worked, I became conscious that I was itching all over my body and after a while I noticed a couple of small lumps on my arm, like mosquito bites. I thought that a mozzie, which are very common in Houston, must have got into the study and started to nibble away at me. I went off to get the insect spray and after giving the room a good dousing, got back to the computer. Minutes later the itching was starting to get really uncomfortable, and I decided to take a shower and wash off the thing that was eating me. My hurried dash into the bedroom caused Carol to wake with a start and she asked me what was wrong. When I explained, she asked me to let her see for herself. As I let my dressing gown slip, she let out an exclamation so loud, that I realised things were worse than

I'd thought. She worried me into the shower cubicle and turned on the cold tap. It was bloody freezing but she insisted that I stay with it, as she banged around in the medicine cupboard. I was now starting to feel really groggy and my head was reeling. I looked down and noticed the whole of my body was covered with hives, the size of 20p pieces. Carol, still ransacking the medicine cabinet, asked me if I was feeling OK but when I went to answer her, no sound came out. My throat had closed and I was struggling to breathe. Suddenly, the shower door burst open and Carol lunged at me, forcing a pill between my lips. "It's antihistamine," she blurted, "That should start to help very quickly."

After a few minutes I was able to talk but my body was still a mass of hives. Clearly I'd had an allergic reaction to something and as Carol drove us to the emergency room, we tried to work out what had caused it. As I had not eaten anything and only drunk a cup of coffee that morning, it was hard to imagine what it could be. Carol asked if I'd taken my blood pressure tablets - and then it dawned on me. I had switched to new pills that morning, as the type I had used in the UK weren't available in the US. Obviously they didn't agree with me; in fact they seriously disagreed with me. In the ER they pumped me full of stuff to overcome the effects and by just after 9 o'clock I was fit enough to be discharged. Fortunately, the location for my pre-op work was in the same building as the ER and as I checked in for my appointment, I apologised for being a few minutes late "only I've been in hospital." The nurse merely smiled and shrugged her shoulders.

Late that evening, with the drama over, I was back to thinking about a holiday. I broached the subject again but Carol's mind was elsewhere. I went onto the Internet and looked at cheaptickets.com and found a trip to Las Vegas for five days and asked Carol for her views. It wasn't her ideal but it seemed to me to be the perfect location for a 'last fling' and she sort of agreed so I said I would book it. With the deed done I said, "Shall we pack?" She looked a bit surprised and asked when we were leaving. "First thing in the morning, I replied.

Our trip to Vegas was exactly what I needed. All the pent-up frustration was overcome as we were better able to enjoy time together without always being reminded of what we would have to face when we returned home. For now we were able to set that aside and enjoy the break. We took in a lot of shows, did a little gambling, although it would hardly rate as more than a flutter on most people's scale, and we saw the sights of this Mecca to excess. We ate and drank well and generally enjoyed the relaxed atmosphere of this surreal world in the desert. Whilst we were there I was able to fulfil my needs, although this had now become a much less important issue than simply being able to spend time together. I thoroughly enjoyed the break and was so glad that we had made the effort, but now it was time to get back to reality. We returned home only three days before the operation. We hadn't spent much time thinking about it while we were away, but now it was the only thing on our minds.

In those last days, the telephone rang off the wall. It appeared as though everyone we knew rang to wish me luck, which was very kind of them. For many, they were unaware of what was involved so I found myself going over the procedure time and again. With each phone call, I could see Carol becoming more distressed as I repeated the procedure for each caller. It was bad enough for her that it had to happen; she certainly didn't want it played out over and over again. Occasionally, she would deal with the call, but in the end she didn't want to speak to or hear from anyone. The day before the operation was particularly tough for her. I was really feeling for her but as I didn't share her concern for my predicament, it was hard to deal with. I was particularly taken aback when she asked what I wanted to happen to my mortal remains if I should die. I tried to laugh it off but this was no laughing matter. For Carol this was hell.

She was concerned about how she would be able to deal with enquiries about me after I'd had the operation. Reading between the lines, she was asking how she could cope if things went badly wrong. She didn't want to deal with a barrage of telephone conversations. I suggested she used the email and one of the last constructive things I did before I went into hospital was to create three email groups on her computer: Friends, family and work, although in practice, one group would have sufficed. It proved to be a great way of informing people of events and, on occasions when the issues become more complex, it was a useful way of sharing the detail, rather than have to go through it with each person individually. This made the telephone conversations more productive and Carol felt better able to deal with them. After I was discharged from hospital, I continued the updates and one of our friends was so taken with them that she commented that I was helping them, rather than them helping me – interesting thought but not true. The emails kept me occupied and focused.

During the weeks leading up to my operation, the bikes had played a crucial role in my fitness regime and my cardio vascular rate (whatever it is) was going up as my weight was coming down. By the time I checked in for my operation I was a full thirty pounds lighter and a whole lot fitter. I felt I'd done a pretty good job and so did the doctor.

# 9
# The Final Cut

On the morning of the operation I was getting dressed when I suddenly realised that it was four months to the day since I'd arrived in the US. It had probably been one of the most eventful four months of my life, and not for the reasons I would have preferred. Now it was about to culminate in being sliced open for a surgical procedure. I wasn't looking forward to it, but knew I had no choice; it had to be done.

We set off in plenty of time, arriving at the hospital just before 9.00 a.m. They were ready for us and took us to a preparation room where I changed into a gown and the nurse fitted a couple of shuttles on the back of my hand, which I presumed were to be used during the procedure. After a while I was prepared for the theatre and the anaesthetist had been round to discuss his part in the performance. He promised to return shortly. Doctor Freidman came by to brief us on how things would progress during the operation. He gave us the glad tidings that if the cancer had spread to the lymph glands, that he wouldn't continue. He then said that if Carol wished to stay in the visitors' room, he would give her an update of how things were going during the operation. Our look obviously told him that we hadn't quite understood – we were still thinking about his previous bombshell. He explained that at various stages he would 'pop out' of the theatre and give Carol a bulletin.

*Brian Turner*

As the visitors' room was quite public, I had visions of him wafting into the room in gown and mask and holding up signs at regular intervals.

'Attention Mrs. Turner. 'Stomach open' - 'lymph nodes in lab' – 'lymph nodes clear' (hopefully) – 'prostate out' – 'scissors missing'.

I sat on the edge of the trolley while the anaesthetist inserted the epidural in my back and down my spine. Not a joyous experience but he assured me that this type of pain control would be beneficial and was worth the early discomfort. I was trying not to concentrate too much on the pain and noticed three ladies, whom I assumed to be theatre nurses, who would be assisting in my mini-drama. As one of them moved away, I could see a vast array of shiny operating implements laid out in a long row. I asked if they were preparing lunch and one of them quipped "Yes! And you're on the menu." By now, the anaesthetist was finishing his work and asked me to lie down on the operating table. As I did so, he said, "Say goodnight."

Well, this was it, I thought. Goodbye prostate – goodbye bladder control – goodbye to glorious erections – goodbye brave worl… and I was gone.

Radical prostate surgery usually lasts two to three hours and mine was the top side of this at nearly four.

## Please Leave The Seat Up

The objective is to completely remove the prostate, as well as the attached seminal vesicles. Two different techniques are used in this type of operation. The method, which Freidman used on me, was called retropubic[8], which is the more common. This involves making an incision from below the navel to the base of the penis. Freidman's first job was to remove some of my pelvic lymph nodes and send them to pathology where they were quick frozen with liquid nitrogen and examined for evidence of cancer. This process is called a pelvic node dissection[9]. (I wonder if he took this opportunity while this was going on, to hold up his first sign in the visitors' room).

Obviously, the results were favourable[10] because he continued with the operation. His next task was to separate the prostate and seminal vesicles from my bladder and rectum and then remove my prostate gland. This was a particularly tricky part of the operation as he had to make a cut through my urethra just above the external sphincter, and another cut just below the internal sphincter at the neck of my bladder. These cuts need to be extremely precise otherwise damage can easily occur. Next, he used a Foley catheter as a guide, to reattach the urethra to the bladder neck using very fine sutures to ensure that the connection was urine-tight. The catheter tube in my bladder ultimately terminated out

---

[8] The alternative technique is the perineal method and involves entry through an incision made between the base of the penis and the rectum.
[9] The medical term for this is a lymphadenectomy.
[10] If the frozen section contains cancer cells, the operation is usually aborted. The presence of cancer in the lymph nodes suggests that the area of the cancer has gone beyond the prostate and therefore, its removal won't free the patient of cancer, but leave him with all the negative side-effects of the surgery.

through my penis and had to remain in place for two weeks, as I was obviously going to be incontinent without my prostate.

My first vision as I woke up was Carol looking down on me and smiling. I took this as a good sign, as this was the first time I'd seen her smile in weeks. I didn't have a clue at that stage, exactly what had happened but if she was happy, then so was I. As I lay there drifting in and out of consciousness, I occasionally wondered if they had done the operation or not. I wasn't yet able to speak to Carol, so I never got to ask her the question. However, for anyone who finds themselves in the same situation, the easiest way to check is to feel your left thigh. If you find a plastic bag attached to it, then good news! That's the catheter, which of course, you will only need if you have had the prostate removed. I'll remember that myself next time I have my prostate removed.

I was aware that Carol had gone, but I was so groggy that all I wanted to do was sleep. I had no idea what time it was, nor did I particularly care. I was safe in my drug-induced state and wanted to stay like that for a while. I wasn't looking forward to the pain, after I regained full consciousness. I continued to drift and realised that I was now in a ward, but beyond that, everything was a blur. Later, I became aware of a lady at the foot of the bed who apologised for waking me. She looked familiar but I couldn't place her, although I wasn't really trying that hard. I asked what the time was and she told me that it was eight o'clock in the evening. I suddenly realised that it was May, a colleague from work, who was kindly bringing some flowers. Apparently, she had intended to leave them on the table and go, but I was awake now and we chatted for a while before she left. However, apart from remembering that she had been, I have absolutely no idea what we talked about. It was a really kind gesture though and one example of so many such actions that would demonstrate that people cared about me and would make me feel very humble over the coming months.

I had been asleep and 'out of it' for the whole day, thanks largely to the epidural. I hadn't had anything to eat or drink, although apparently, when I first woke up, I'd asked the nurse for a pint of beer: She wasn't amused. During the evening, the nurse came round a few times and moistened my lips with ice, but apart from that, I had no other basic needs to be dealt with. The bag, which was firmly strapped to my leg, was obviously taking care of my toiletry requirements and I was reasonably comfortable.

When the nurse did my vitals at about midnight, she asked me if I had any gas. I learnt that this was the American way of asking if I'd farted. I told her that I hadn't and feeling quite indignant was tempted to add that if she was able to smell one, it must be hers. She put my chart back on the end of the bed and told me that it wasn't good. She said, "You need to have gas," and turned away, leaving me to contemplate her invitation to have a rip-roaring fart. As most people who know me will testify, breaking wind has never been something with which I have ever found difficulty, nor have I been too coy in sharing it with others if the matter arose. In fact, some might even suggest it was one of my core competencies. But now that my big moment had arrived, I was unable to muster even the merest whiff. It was as if breaking wind had suddenly been lost from my array of bodily functions.

Suddenly, an almighty blast reverberated around the room, which sadly didn't come from me. For the first time since I'd been admitted to the ward, I realised that I was sharing the room with someone else, and he wasn't behind the door when it came to putting on a performance for the nurse. Over and over, his rear end trumpeted in relentless triumph. If there were prizes for 'having gas', this guy was about to receive the lifetime achievement award. The nurse had requested that I 'have gas' as well and I was determined not to let her down. But my gas was not forthcoming, so I tried to get some sleep again and see what developed.

At about 2.00 a.m. the nurse was round again and I mentioned that I was starting to feel a lot of pain. "Any gas?" she demanded. "No," I groaned, "Just pain." "Well you need gas," she reiterated, shaking her head in dismay, and left me to it once more. By four o'clock I was in so much pain that I pressed my night bell. The nurse came in and I told her I needed more pain control and asked if she could increase the flow on the epidural. That was clearly not within her remit. Instead she insisted on turning me over and repositioned me with my knees drawn up to my stomach. I couldn't imagine how that would help the pain; I was in agony and I told her so. She referred me to a chart on the wall. It contained a line of ten cartoon faces; the one at the extreme left had a big beaming smile, while the one at the far right looking totally miserable with tears pouring down his face and sweat beads emitting from the top of his head. "How bad is your pain on the scale of smiley faces?" she asked. I told her it was pretty bad. "Is it ten?" she prompted. I told that it wasn't that bad, otherwise "I would be screaming - trust me." I confirmed that it was about eight. "OK!" she said, picking up my chart again, "eight on the smiley faces," and wrote something down. In between my stabbing pains, I had a vision of her drawing a round miserable face on my chart.

I lay there feeling sorry for myself and trying to endure the pain. Within a few minutes, I could feel the gas welling up and suddenly it was out. It was long and loud and certainly gave the guy in the next bed a run for his money. If this was about to turn into a competition, I had started with a good solid opening shot and would soon be catching up fast. After a relatively short period, I was starting to neck into lead position, which wasn't too difficult as the other guy hadn't produced any gas for quite a while and appeared to have retired defeated. Meanwhile, I was home and dry and hopefully impressing the hell out of the nurse. However, my opponent, who had now started to moan loudly, interrupted my smug satisfaction. I was thinking of asking him if he was OK, but we hadn't been formally introduced and you know what we Brits are like for formality. Unable to rely on any help from me, he pressed the night bell and seconds later the nurse came in.

"Arghhh! Arrrghh!" he was yelling at the top of his voice, as she approached his bed. "What number on the smiley faces?" she snapped at him. "Ten – ten – ten – ten," he kept repeating and he did sound pretty distressed. After a bit of commotion and lots of activity behind the curtain, I heard an almighty fart and my neighbour let out an "Oooohhaaarrhh" of great relief. After a bit more activity, the nurse left. As he had been invading my ears with so much fuss, I felt more inclined to introduce myself and said to him, "You sounded a bit rough there for a while, mate." He pulled back the curtain so that we got our first sight of each other and he said, "I've just had my prostate removed and I had a terrible build up of gas." I knew the feeling. We spent the next little while swapping notes and Allan, who was about seventy, told me that, when this type of operation is undertaken, a large amount of air enters the body, which then has to be disgorged by breaking wind. Little wonder that the nurse had been urging me on earlier in the night, but thankfully we were both now playing 'Trumpet Voluntary' in unison, quickly moving down the smiley faces chart to 'Mr. Happy'.

Sometime later, the nurse came back and didn't ask either of us about the gas. I'm sure her nostrils were getting the message that we were both doing fine in that department. She brought Allan his breakfast but looked across to me and said, "You'll get something later." I asked her for some water as I was parched, but she gave me a cup of ice instead, telling me that I couldn't have water just yet, although I could use the crushed ice to moisten my lips. I did it a couple of times but it did nothing to quench my raging thirst, so I put the cup under the blankets and held it against my body to melt it. Within ten minutes I was able to get the drink that I so badly craved and which she had denied me.

Carol arrived and I was so pleased to see her smiling. Hopefully, she was feeling a lot happier about things, now that the surgery was over. Next time the nurse came by, she told me that I had to get up and walk around this morning. Blimey, I thought. I have nothing to eat or drink (well not that she knew about) and she expects me to gallop around like a racehorse. However, trying to be the model patient, I did her bidding and when she helped me up, I sat on the edge of the bed for a few minutes, and then I stood up – and fell back down again. The room seemed to be spinning and I felt sick. She insisted I got back into bed and this time I was in complete agreement with her. "We'll try again later," she said as she tucked me up. Much later if I had anything to do with it.

During the morning the anaesthetist who had performed during my operation came to visit. He removed my epidural and asked the nurse to give me pain-killing pills as the effects of the anaesthetic wore off. As it turned out, the pain never got any worse and I only had one tablet before deciding that I could manage without them. A bit later, Doctor Freidman called by to see how I was doing and we sat chatting for a while before he went back to the operating theatre to deny some other unfortunate soul the use of his prostate. I was impressed. I hadn't expected to see the surgeon at all, thinking that he would be present only during the operation, but he had already spent time preparing me for chop, and now he was here again after the event. I was feeling like I was getting the royal treatment.

*Brian Turner*

Lunchtime arrived and a tray of goodies was placed in front of me. The note on the tray said 'As you were asleep, we have made a selection from the menu on your behalf'. It also stated that I was on a liquid diet. Now, I've had liquid lunches before but they usually consisted of Wadsworth 6X or a good pint of Bass, but as I cast my eyes over the tray, I realised they meant something completely different. There was soup, a yogurt and a number of other things which, I have to confess, at that moment, looked even more exciting than a pint of beer, although when I started eating, I realised that I had absolutely no appetite whatsoever. After only a few spoonfuls of soup, I felt like I'd eaten a banquet and therefore decided to call it a day.

I had a visit from a couple of colleagues later in the afternoon. I don't know how much sense I made during our chat, but after a while I was so tired, I really wanted them to leave me alone in order that I could have a snooze. Later, when I tried to recall the conversation, I could barely remember anything at all, but it had been good to see them, especially as they brought me some books to read. I was just dozing off again when a deliveryman carrying a basket the size of a dustbin walked in. He placed it on the floor and I could see that it was overflowing with plants and flowers. This was a present from all the folks at the office and I'd never seen anything quite like it before. Then I thought, well after all, this is Texas – and everything is bigger in Texas.

Towards the evening, Doctor Nash looked in. He apologised for not having had a chance to chat with me before the operation, but he wanted to assure me that he was there for 'the main event'. "I wouldn't have missed it for the world," he said. "We've all been very interested in your case and I was keen to be in on the action." I was glad he was there. Although I hadn't seen him since the biopsy, somehow, I felt a degree of sentimentality, with him being the guy who had prepared me for the news. He had such a gentlemanly style, in stark contrast to Freidman's 'in yer face' approach. He asked if I'd been able to take a walk during the day. When I told him about the aborted attempt he said that I should try hard tomorrow. "After all, we want to get you home quickly don't we?" he said, smiling.

Having had a good night's sleep, by the next morning I was feeling much better and ready for my breakfast, although once again, my appetite let me down. Carol came in early and I was glad to see her and to be able to spend time chatting with her now that I was 'compos mentis'. She helped me to get out of bed and take a few steps around the ward, before helping me to the armchair, where I sat for a couple of hours. It was good to be up and about again. Doctor Freidman called in again and was glad to see me sitting up. He told me a lot more about the operation, and in particular, that my prostate had been full of cancer. "It certainly was a good one," he confided. "We don't see many like that in the US." I was unsure whether he expected me to be pleased or disappointed, but either way, I was glad it was out.

Later that day I had a lesson from the nurse about how to empty my catheter. There was a toilet in the ward, and although it was only about ten yards away from my bed, the first time I walked it, it felt like I'd run a marathon. While I was in there, the nurse told me to take a shower. It was pretty tricky with all the paraphernalia that I had attached to me, so I was glad that she stayed around to provide help, although I'm sure it must have looked really amusing with her holding the catheter as I shampooed my hair. Each of these things was getting me another step nearer to going home and I was anticipating being out by Monday morning, so long as I kept making good progress. By dinner that night I was back on solids and enjoyed a meal of chicken and two veg; although my appetite was still struggling with the size of the Texas portions.

On Sunday morning, I didn't wait for the nurse to come round. I got up, emptied the catheter and had a shower, finding a novel way of dealing with the catheter as I did so, by hooking it up over the shower head. After putting on a clean pair of pyjamas, rather than the hospital gown, I now started to walk up and down outside my room, as if to demonstrate how well I was doing. Finally, I needed to rest, so I sat in my chair and listened to some music. I was feeling pretty good and much more human. The bag of pee sitting on the floor beside me was the only thing that gave a lie to my wellness. I was surprised to see Doctor Nash at about eight-thirty and asked him if this was a normal workday for him. He told me he lived locally and had popped in to see how I was doing. I was impressed; not only by this action, but by all the care and treatment I'd received so far. I was made to feel like an important customer and these little touches were quite humbling.

Thinking back to the news that Freidman had given

me the previous day about the amount of cancer in my prostate, I asked Doctor Nash how long he thought I'd had the cancer. He sat thoughtfully and said, "Hard to say, but it's likely that it's been there for a number of years." I was surprised and as I sat contemplating the news he added, "Looking at the condition of it, we couldn't have left it any longer, otherwise you would have been in serious trouble." I asked exactly what he meant and he said that although the lymph nodes had been clear, in another three months, it would have been a very different story.

Bloody hellfire; did I feel like Mr Lucky. I realised, in an instant, the implications of what he had said although I'm not sure he knew just how profound this was. If I had not come to America, I would ultimately have died from my cancer. It was as clear as that. With a Gleason of 8 the cancer was likely to be doubling in size every few months and if the prostate was 'full' when they took it out, then the DRE that had triggered Doctor Epstein to refer me to Doctor Nash, had saved my life. As no such screening process is available in the UK, and I hadn't been experiencing any noticeable problems with my bladder, there would have been no chance of it being detected before it was too late. This was indeed a defining moment for me and one which I will always remember. I vowed there and then that I would be an advocate for DRE and PSA testing in the UK and would be urging all my male friends and colleagues over fifty to insist on being checked out.

Onto more mundane matters, Doctor Nash asked if I'd been shown how to use a day catheter (also known as a leg catheter), which I hadn't. As he left, he said he would ask the nurse to show me how to use one. Then, almost as an afterthought, he said, "Do you feel well enough to go home today?" I beamed a smile at him and said, "You bet."

Twenty minutes later I was packing up my personal belongings, having had the leg catheter demo a few minutes earlier. I was fully mobile and raring to go – home. I was surprised that Carol had not been in by now and called her on the phone. She said that she had decided to visit a bit later today but when I told her that I was packed and waiting for her, she was surprised and delighted that I was being discharged. She said, "I'm on my way."

Whilst I was waiting, I took the opportunity to thank all the nursing staff for looking after me so well. My hospital experience had been excellent and so it was with a tinge of sadness that I was leaving and I was quite nervous as the nurse escorted me out to Carol's car. Even though it was the middle of December, it was a warm sunny day and I was looking forward to being home again.

## 10
## Good to be Home

Carol made sure I was comfortable and nursed me with undivided attention. I didn't want for much; the first few days were taken up with sleeping, eating small portions of soft food, drinking and sleeping. In fact, although sleeping was my main activity for the first week or so, I found I could only ever stay asleep for a period of 2 hours. Often I would go to bed at 8.00 p.m. and be up pacing around at 10.00. My sleep pattern was so erratic that Carol slept in the spare room for the first month in order to get enough rest to keep her going the next day, nursing me. She tells me that I was a good patient but I think she is being more than generous. She seemed to spend her whole day looking after me. I was conscious that she was watching like a hawk. I would be watching TV and feel her eyes burning into me. When I looked up she asked if I was OK. Of course I was OK. With this level of attention, if I were to have a sudden heart attack, she would have caught me before I had time to hit the floor.

On some occasions, such constant concern was a drain and I suggested that she went out for a spot of retail therapy. Over the next few months I think she must have visited almost every shop in Houston, judging by the bags and boxes she brought back each time. I was amazed some weeks later when we went for a drive. It appeared that she had done the Texas version of "The Knowledge". There wasn't a road she didn't know or the location of a shop that she couldn't give exact directions to. Maybe I'd overdone getting her out of the house so often.

I was scheduled to have my stitches removed 7 days after my release from hospital. In fact, they were not stitches but large staples; about twelve of them running from my navel to the base of my penis. I certainly wasn't looking forward to having them removed. It was with great trepidation that I presented myself to Freidman's office, but I needn't have worried. When he took them out he was quicker than Michael Schumacher approaching the chequered flag.

He asked how I was getting on at home and I mentioned to him that I was having cramp during the night. He immediately instructed the nurse to set up an ultra sound on my leg and turned to me saying, "Don't leave the hospital today until you've had the ultrasound. This could be a blood clot and we don't want you dying on the way home." Hear, hear to that I thought. Anyway, I went for the ultrasound as instructed but it proved to be nothing to worry about. Thank goodness for that, I had enough drama to contend with, without dying on the way home.

Having to use a catheter is neither good nor bad – it's just a bit fiddly. As a convenience aid it's pretty inconvenient, having to empty it every couple of hours. Luckily, the manufacturers had had enough forethought to have a day bag and a night bag. A day bag is similar in construction to the night type only smaller. It was strapped to my left leg so that when I was fully dressed, it was not easily detectable and it provided for a lot more mobility, although I had to remember to empty it frequently. The day bag could hold about a litre, whereas the night bag held about three litres, which meant I didn't have to keep leaping out of bed during the night. Not that I was in much of a position to leap anywhere at that time. The ritual cleaning and changing of bags was a bit irritating and I found the whole thing somewhat undignified, so I was looking forward to having it removed, especially as we had friends flying in from the UK on 28th December to share the New Year festivities with us. Obviously, as you will have realised by now if you have been following the pattern of my thinking throughout, I'd given no thought to what would come after the catheter was removed. I was still dealing with things one step at a time and I was certainly keen to get rid of the 'old bag'. It was only the evening before I was due to have it taken away that I started to consider how tricky life might be without it. I was back in Freidman's office on Boxing Day, (a working day in the US), and I was about to find out.

Before he got down to business, he talked me through how I was to manage the process of regaining control of my bladder. This was apparently going to be achieved with the help of a 'Doctor Arnold', who had developed pelvic muscle exercises or Kegel (kay-gull) exercises as they were called. The idea is to strengthen the pelvic floor muscles[11] and use them to control the bladder now that the prostate was no longer able to fulfil the role. These muscles contract and relax to control the opening and closing of the urethral sphinc-

---
[11] The medical name for these muscles is the 'pubococcygeus' muscles.

ters, the muscles that give urinary control. While these muscles remained weak, I would continue to leak urine. Freidman informed me that through regular exercise, I might be able to build up their strength and endurance and, hopefully, regain my bladder control.

The following is an extract of the fact sheet he gave me to read and develop my proficiency in pelvic floor muscle control. I understand that this is the method women rely on for controlling the bladder, as clearly, they don't come equipped with a prostate.

*Begin by locating the muscles to be exercised:*

1. *As you begin urinating, try to stop or slow the urine without tensing the muscles of your legs, buttocks, or abdomen. It is very important not to use these other muscles, because only the pelvic floor muscles help with bladder control.*

2. *When you are able to slow or stop the stream of urine, you have located the correct muscles. Feel the sensation of the muscles pulling inward and upward.*

    *Helpful hint: Squeeze in the rectal area to tighten the anus as if trying not to pass gas. You will be using the correct muscles.*

If you have been keeping up with me, you will have also been trying to locate the correct muscle as you read the instructions, and are preparing to exercise along

## Please Leave The Seat Up

with me.

*Now you are ready to exercise regularly. Tighten and relax the sphincter muscles as rapidly as you can. Next contract the sphincter muscle and hold to a count of 3, then RELAX completely before the next contraction. In the beginning, check yourself frequently by looking in the mirror or by placing a hand on your abdomen and buttocks to ensure that you do not feel your belly, thigh, or buttock muscles move. If there is movement, continue to experiment until you have isolated just the muscles of the pelvic floor.*

*Make pelvic muscle exercises a part of your daily routine: You must do them regularly on a lifetime basis. Use daily routines such as watching TV, reading, stopping at traffic lights, and waiting in the grocery checkout line as cues to perform a few exercises.*

I found myself doing the exercises in the strangest of places. People give you the oddest of looks when you're trying to clench your cheeks together. It brings a whole new meaning to being 'Anal retentive'.

It laid out some other handy hints, which were a sign of how I was to conduct my life from here on in.

When you have the urge to urinate try the following:

- *Stop what you're doing and sit down or stand still and remain quiet. Relax you body by taking a few deep breaths.*

- *Do some Kegel squeezes quickly 3 or 4 times without relaxing.*
- *Concentrate hard on suppressing the urge to urinate and wait until the urge passes or subsides.*
- *Once the urge has subsided, walk at a regular pace to the bathroom. Don't run. Continue to do the Kegel squeezes as you walk.*

When Freidman had finished his run-through on the Kegel routine, he asked me if I had any questions. I said that I had understood it all and very nearly told him I thought it would be "a piece of piss" but simply assured him that it was "all very clear thank you."

After the chat he removed the catheter so quickly, it took me by surprise. He urged me to have a practiced pee, which was successful and appeared to delight him no end. He handed me a small pad and suggested that I might need it to protect myself from any leakage on my trip home. What he should have said is 'you might need this to protect yourself until you get to the toilet just down the hall.' Because by the time I had reached the car, the pad, my underpants and trousers were soaked and I had pee running down my legs. Apart from being bloody uncomfortable, it was extremely distressing. If I'd given this any thought beforehand, I might have been better prepared.

As soon as we arrived home, Carol headed off to the nearest pharmacy to get something to help with the problem, while I hovered between sitting on a chair piled with old towels and making a run for the loo. Eventually, I found the toilet a safer bet and decided

# Please Leave The Seat Up

to stay put until Carol's return. Unfortunately, I forgot to take a book in with me and, being reluctant to make another excursion from the safety of the porcelain, stayed perched on the WC until she returned. Luckily the shops were only a couple of miles away.

Everyone knows that the US is the ultimate consumer society and I was even more pleased by this than usual when it came to dealing with my incontinence. Through my wife's work with the elderly, she had told me how difficult it was to get incontinence pads from the local chemist in the UK. Well, no such problem in the US. We didn't even need to rely on the chemist's; they also stocked them in supermarkets. At the last count, they had over twenty different types with sizes ranging from 'oops, a bit of a dribble' to 'Watch Out! - Tidal wave'. However, in those early days, I really needed a size, which they didn't yet stock: 'Niagara Falls.' Nevertheless, I feel sure that they'll soon spot this gap in the market and plug it with another complete range, including pads, which emit a perfume of 'fragrant rose petals in the early morning dew'.

Fortunately, Carol soon returned, armed with an array of pads and I was so *'relieved'* to get my hands on them. I was sure that this was the end of my problems and I could get on with my Kegel exercises. No doubt I would be back to work in a few weeks.

Early that evening, I was sitting on the toilet yet again, and as I stood up, I noticed some blood in the pan. I wasn't too panicky but called for Carol to come and give her expert opinion. She didn't need to look in the pan to know that all was not well. As she got to the door she let out a gasp and clasping her hands to her mouth said, "Oh my God. What have you done?"

Done? Done? I hadn't done anything apart from what was becoming a familiar and regular event. "I've had a pee and there is some blood in the water. Do you think the doctor damaged something when he removed the catheter?"

"Your stitches," she shouted as she pointed to my stomach.

I didn't understand what she was saying. I'd had my stitches (or staples) out a week ago. But as I looked down I realised why she was getting in such a state. My operation wound had opened along three quarters of its length and blood was flowing freely down my body and dripping into a neat red pool at my feet. Carol tried the best she could to administer first aid by wrapping a large bandage around me in an attempt to hold things together, but she was fighting a losing battle with my rotund stomach. Very soon we were making a mad dash to the ER with Carol at the wheel, playing dodgems with the rush-hour traffic while I tried to hold my stomach together and stem the bleeding. Obviously, I was a priority case, but not before the hospital administrators had checked that I had the means to pay for the treatment. I sat and bled on the waiting room floor while they checked my insurance details. However, once they had completed the paperwork, they lost no time in getting me into a cubicle and lying down. I was glad I had remembered to pick up my insurance card as I left the house. I hate to imagine what they may have done if I'd forgotten to bring it in the drama of the moment.

By the time the doctor arrived, the bleeding had stopped but I still had a gaping slit in my stomach as if I'd been attacked by a mad axe-man. He arranged for someone to apply a 'wet and dry' dressing to my wound and bound me up with a stretch bandage. Before leaving he instructed me to see Doctor Freidman in his office the following morning. After spending several hours in the hospital, Carol drove us home at a more measured pace than we had arrived. As we retraced our route I was half expecting to see the road littered with wrecked cars that had become casualties in our earlier journey. We reflected on the day that had started off as a milestone in my recovery and had turned out to be a huge setback. One thing's for sure. It had been pretty eventful.

I was dreading my visit to the doctor the next morning. The wound area was still tender from the operation and the previous night's events had compounded the discomfort. I really wasn't looking forward to having another lot of stitches – or, worse still, staples. I had visions of the doctor picking up the Rexel from his desk and punching holes into my stomach to knit the thing together. Freidman was surprised to see me in his office at the crack of dawn and even more surprised to see the gaping hole in my stomach. To my relief, he didn't have his trusty staple gun swinging in his holster. Instead he decided that the 'wet and dry' dressing would be the appropriate way to deal with it and asked Carol to come close in order that he could instruct her on the procedure. He started by saying, "This is what you will need to do," at which point she shook her head and turned up her nose in horror. She was trying to let him know that she was unable to do this, preferring to leave it to experts. He didn't respond, but carried on demonstrating and instructing her on the process. When he had finished he told her that she needed to go to the pharmacy and purchase bottles of saline wash and Hydrogen Peroxide – and plenty of gauze dressing and cotton wool. Clearly, he was not entertaining her protestations, taking the view that, 'he's yours – deal with it'. Now in a more conciliatory frame of mind, she asked him how often she would need to dress it.

"Three or four times a day until the wound has completely knitted together; it should take about a month."

So I was feeling pleased at not having to be stapled together again and Carol was mortified at the thought of having to dress the wound, even once, let alone four times a day for a month, although she never complained. As we headed back home, I leant over and squeezed her knee and as she looked across I said, "Sorry." She smiled back and I could see she was already coming to terms with it.

This was turning into a game of 'Challenge Anika' only this was 'Challenge Brian.' Not only was my stomach trying spontaneously to unzip itself, but I also had a bladder which had developed a mind of its own and regardless of any efforts with the Kegel exercises, which incidentally strained at my wound, I had no control. Whenever I took my Paddy-Pads off, I would instantly pee where I stood. When I was lying down it was less of a problem but as soon as I stood up my bladder would empty. I had become the urine equivalent of the 'Cinzano man'. I would pee 'any time, any place, anywhere'. Consequently, I remained padded up at all times except when I was in the shower. After only a few days of facing up to the situation of constantly peeing myself, I had to tackle my next unexpected challenge – NAPPY RASH.

It's obvious really but I'd not given it a thought. If your wedding tackle is immersed in urine for any length of time, nappy rash will occur. Ask any baby and he will tell you; well he would if he could talk. Nevertheless, he communicates it well enough by yelling. I have noticed that when baby boys get nappy rash their testicles shrivel up like prunes. So how might that feel in an adult man? Well let me tell you. It's bloody agony! Within a matter of days my testicles had shrivelled beyond the size and shape of walnuts and were shrinking as fast as they could to try and extricate themselves from this hostile environment. As they continued to shrink the pain was more intense and there was no let-up.

Carol, who by now was almost living at the pharmacy, purchased every ointment she could find for 'diaper rash' but to no avail. I was getting in a bit of a state, not knowing where I hurt the most. Then Carol suggested that we try the good old stand-by, Vaseline. I walloped a handful of that around my equipment and the cooling sensation alone was a bit of a relief. Every time I went to the loo - which incidentally was a bit of a pointless exercise as the contents of my bladder were usually in my pad - I would give my testicles another good greasing with the Vaseline. In a few days life was bearable again and it continued to improve over the next several days.

As I lay in bed one afternoon, having my usual nap, I started to think how I might improve things even more. I couldn't wait until I qualified for my 'Kegel proficiency badge' as that could take months. No, instead, I needed to find a better method of keeping myself dry. They say that necessity is the mother of invention. How true that is. As I lay there I concentrated on how I might re-stack the odds so that they were more in my favour. Over the course of an hour I developed a strategy. Firstly, I would remain sitting, or lying whenever possible, preferably in close proximity to the toilet. Then whenever my bladder showed signs of needing to be emptied, I would get to the loo as quickly as I could, giving me the best chance of getting some of it down the pan rather than in my underpants. Finally, and this was the masterstroke, I would do an 'Eleanor Rigby': by keeping a jar by my bed.

When I got up I told Carol of the plan and we moved the furniture around to suit. That night, as I got into bed, I placed an empty Robertson's jam jar on the bedside cabinet. As I dropped off to sleep I felt sure that the Golly was smiling at me. At about one o'clock I woke up and grabbed for the jar, putting it over myself as I stood up to go to the loo. Eureka! Instant success: In one stroke I'd reduced the problem from all to nothing. I toddled over to the toilet and let out the remaining dregs then emptied and washed the jar. I climbed back into bed and for the first time my pad was still bone dry: An excellent result.

The next afternoon, I awoke from my nap and my mind was back to the previous night's success. Rather than feeling satisfied that I'd come up with a great discovery, I was already thinking of refinements to my strategy: One that would allow me to venture out of the house without the usual worry and the carrier bag full of nappies. I concluded that if the jar worked so well at night, it might form part of the solution during the day. However, I was struggling to imagine how I might walk around with a jar in my underpants without people noticing. Obviously, some men are well endowed but I doubted if even the luckiest of them was ever this size. Undeterred, I continued to mull it over until I came up with an idea for the ultimate 'device'. I worked the details out in my mind, thankful that the vast amount of money the government had spent on my engineering training in the Royal Navy all those years ago had, at last, come into play, just when I needed it most. But now I had to try and convey my idea into words so that I could brief Carol on my exact requirements. After all, she would be the one who would have to source the item for me.

As I talked her through it, using sketches to assist in my explanation, she assured me that she now had a clear picture. She delved into cupboards and rattled around in drawers, eventually finding some vessels, which were close to the model I had in mind. I tried them out but none of them were ideal, although they helped us to refine the exact requirements. She went off to the shops and within the hour had returned with two likely containers. One was good but proved to be a little uncomfortable. The second was perfect and would become the 'device', which I used for the next few weeks while I continued with my Kegel exercises. It was a baby's feeding bottle; approximately eight inches long with a 35-degree bend about halfway along its length. The neck, in which I fitted a small rubber ring, was just large enough for my penis to fit through and was a neat enough fit that it didn't rub when I walked. It was kept in place by my padded knickers and the angle of the bottle allowed it to sit comfortably between my legs without sticking out, although I'm not sure it would have passed the Lycra shorts test.

From then on I was in clover. During the day I would wear the bottle and at night I used the jar. I felt sure that all men who undergo a prostate operation must be faced with the same problems and wished I had been able to speak to people to find out how they had overcome them, rather than learn the hard way. After a few weeks, my Kegel exercises were paying off and I started to regain some of the control. Later still I stopped relying on the 'device', only using it if I went out for lengthy periods. However, I now had to tackle a more routine issue. My wife, like most women I suspect, had spent most of our married life asking me to put the toilet seat down after I had used it. With my need to attend to toilet matters with some urgency, I now had to remind her on a daily basis to "Please Leave the Seat Up".

I found it ironic that before I had the operation most of my thoughts had been about how I would come to terms with being impotent. In reality, I should have been concerned with the incontinence. Little did I realise that dealing with that problem would dwarf everything else in the months after I came out of hospital.

## 11
## Messing with my Hormones

Carol continued to dress the wound four times a day as I lay there, helpless and fully compliant. I think she enjoyed that bit as it was a rarity for her to have me under her full control. She would lay an old towel around my groin to prevent any of the saline or hydrogen-peroxide from running down onto my 'most sensitive' bits, which did actually happen once in the early days and I nearly hit the roof. Thankfully, the use of the towel ensured there wasn't a repeat performance. Even though I was now impotent, I was quite keen to retain my equipment in the right place even if it was only for display purposes. After a few weeks we noticed that the towel was starting to fall apart. The liquids had caused it to rot and it was full of holes. I was now even more glad that she had used it as protection – what would I look like with holey testicles? Answers on a postcard please.

Following the removal of my prostate, a more thorough examination of the cells was carried out in the pathology laboratory. The purpose of this was to establish precisely the location and extent of the tumour and to determine whether the cancer had been confined within the prostate capsule or whether it had spread into the surrounding pelvic cavity and seminal vesicles. To carry out this test, the pathologist coats the outside of the prostate and surrounding tissue with India ink. He then cuts it into thin slices, mounts it in paraffin blocks and places it in a preservative liquid overnight before examining it under a microscope. If he sees that all the edges are clear of ink, it is likely that all of the cancer has been removed. However, if cancer cells are at the edge of the India ink, then the scalpel has cut through cancer, and the operation has not been entirely successful in eradicating the cancer.

The pathology can also determine the Gleason score more accurately at this stage. The pathological Gleason score is rarely lower than the clinical score. Following the pathology testing, my (clinical) Gleason score of 4+4 was re-rated to 5+4, giving an overall Gleason reading of 9. Freidman had been right to be concerned about the aggressiveness of the cancer and it appears that it had been removed not a moment too soon. So much for a score of 5 being a rarity: Obviously not so in my case. This result was enough to have Freidman looking for more information as to the extent of which my cancer had moved outside of the prostate and to know more about how the cancer was developing in the area around my now-discarded prostate. However, he already had enough information to decide that I needed further treatment and he outlined the next steps to us.

1. Immediately undergo a bone scan to check for any cancer cells elsewhere in the area. Review the results of the scan within ten days.

2. Start a two years' course of hormone 'shots' or as we say in the UK, injections, to chemically 'castrate' me.

3. Concurrent with the 'shots', start a course of hormone pills to finally deal with (as he put it) 'the

little blighters', which are danced around in the area of my prostate.

4. Carry out radiation therapy to blast the free cancer cells. This would start in six to ten weeks, once I'd got better control of my bladder.

Before I left Freidman's office, I made an appointment with his nurse to return in ten days to have my first 'shot'. This was the earliest appointment we could arrange, as it had to be approved by my insurance company before it could be ordered.

A few days later I was back at the hospital for a bone scan. I was told to report at eight o'clock in the morning, having fasted from ten the night before. As the nurse led me into the consulting room, I was a little concerned to see a container on his desk with radiation warning stickers all over it. I was even more concerned when he opened it and took out a large hypodermic, which was full of a yellow liquid; the hypodermic primed and ready for action. As he stuck it in my arm he explained that this would now whiz around my body and react with any cancer cells. I was to come back in four hours, after the stuff had had time to work. As I left the office I caught sight of the sign on the door: 'Nuclear Medicine'. Blimey, I thought, it's hardly rocket science. But then again, this is Houston so maybe it is – 'Er, Okay Houston, we have a problem.'

I was now desperate for a cup of coffee and the nurse had told me that I could eat and drink if I wanted to. I wanted to all right but he also told me that I couldn't have any dairy products before the scan, so Starbucks was still on hold. Suffering from caffeine deficiency, I wandered around for four hours waiting for the injection to do its stuff and wondering what was going on inside my body. Every now and then I would check my skin to see if I was starting to glow. I was somewhat disappointed to find that I wasn't and kept expecting to see someone moving in to check me with a Geiger counter at any moment.

At the allotted time I was back at the 'Nuclear Medicine' office and shown to an examination table. I explained to the nurse that I was still incontinent and asked if I should take my pads off and lie on a towel or something. He told me just to keep the pads on and handed me a robe. After donning the robe I hopped – well, okay - I gently climbed onto the table and found myself lying under this large machine. The nurse lowered it until it was hovering just above my body and told me to lie very still while he carried out the scan. As the machine whirred into action, I realised that I was in fact under a gigantic photocopying machine, although this one took half an hour to do a single pass.

When I had been completely Xeroxed, the nurse came over and told me that he had to do it again as there appeared to be some massive clouding around my pelvis. I asked him if it could be the incontinence knickers that I was wearing.

"Are they wet?" he asked.

I felt like shouting, "Of course they're wet, you bloody fool. I'm incontinent." But I simply smiled and said, "Yes, I'm afraid they are."

He suggested that I take the knickers off and lie on a towel for the next one. Now, didn't I suggest that earlier, I thought as I dropped my pants and lay back on the table? This time the result was satisfactory. I got dressed and left.

Hormonal therapy is sometimes used as a primary treatment of prostate cancer, particularly in older men. It's also a major treatment for metastatic disease, which is why Freidman deemed it necessary in my case. The therapy works by shutting down the production of testosterone through a process known as androgen deprivation. That is to say that it 'starves' androgen-dependent cells. The most common method of hormone therapy is through injections of leutenizing hormone-releasing hormone agonist (LH-RH).

The doctor had opted for this method in my case and had prescribed Lupron[12] injections at four monthly intervals and I had my first one – in the hip – during the third week in January. It was supposed to be earlier but apparently my insurance company was taking a long time to sanction payment. Eager to get on with it, I told the nurse that I would pay if it would speed things up. However, when she told me that each shot was $2100, I decided to wait for the insurance company to get their act together.

---

[12] The equivalent drug in the UK is Zoladex

## Please Leave The Seat Up

At the start of a course of Lupron, testosterone levels usually increase dramatically and soon after that, sex drive is lost for the duration of the treatment. I don't know if my testosterone level rose dramatically or not, but my wedding tackle was not aware of any change, remaining as moribund as it had since the day of my operation. I think this must only apply to men who don't have the operation first. It does sound a bit like a sexual roller coaster though. Anyway, it takes about ten weeks before the testosterone decreases to the levels of surgical castration, although, from my point of view, such a delay is worthwhile. The alternative is simply too awful to contemplate. It brings tears to my eyes just to think about it. Some weeks after I started the course of injections, I realised that the castration was complete, as I'd stopped having any thoughts in the sex department whatsoever. I often wondered what a Eunuch thought about and now I knew. Anything… Anything at all - except sex!

The side effects of the hormone treatment include hot flushes and fatigue and I had them both. It's not a great deal of fun to sit in the chair feeling absolutely knackered, while at the same time, breaking out in a sweat every few minutes, but I felt that it must be doing its job.

Unfortunately, the injections on their own are not sufficient to kill all of the cancer cells, as other hormones are produced by the adrenal glands, and continue to grow without androgens. In order to overcome this problem, the doctor had prescribed the anti-androgen Casodex, in pill form. Anti-androgens work by blocking the testosterone from changing into dihydrotestosterone (DHT). These agents are used in combination with LH-RH to achieve what is called a total androgen blockade.

By the time I returned home from my bone scan, Carol had been to the pharmacy to get a month's supply of the Casodex pills. As she waved them in my direction she said, "Do you know how much these were?" Obviously I didn't, but I knew she was about to tell me. Apparently, the pharmacist had enquired how she intended to pay for them. She thought it an odd question and said 'Cash?"

He said, "That's fine but you do realise that it will be four hundred and eighty dollars."

"Four hundred and eighty dollars for a months worth of pills," I exclaimed. "We'll be bankrupt in a few weeks." I soon calmed down again when she explained that she had ascertained from the pharmacist that our medical insurance would reimburse most of the cost and we only had to contribute $20 a month. What a relief!

I was still working on my pelvic wall exercises and now I was having my body filled with female hormones. I started to wonder if the doctors were trying to turn me into a woman. I was watching out for the early signs and was soon aware of my breasts getting larger and my nipples becoming sore. As the chemical castration started to take effect, my penis began to shrink and finally retracted so much that it was flush to my body, making it difficult to use the toilet without sitting down. I was hoping that the hormones wouldn't move me too far towards womanhood, otherwise I might start to lose all sense of reasoned logic and go out on long shopping trips for nothing in particular, returning empty handed and feeling that I'd had a good day out. My worst fear was that I would wake up one morning and open my wardrobe to find 40 pairs of shoes ... and not being able to decide which pair to wear.

The hormone treatment was certainly kicking in big time and I was starting to notice that my emotions were always on the surface. I would have to put up with these changes for the duration of the treatment. It was going to be long time before I was back to my normal self once more.

## 12
## Them Bones, Them Bones

With the hormone treatment underway, strange though it may seem, I was now looking forward to starting the radiation therapy. It wasn't because I was a glutton for punishment, but I felt that I was on a roll and getting on with the radiation would be one step closer to recovery. At my recent appointment, Freidman had suggested that it would start within six to eight weeks and I was anxious to get it done and out of the way as soon as possible. When we saw him again to get the results of the bone scan, I was hoping that he would say, "You're **'Go'** for radiation treatment." I reasoned that if we could get this started soon, I could get back to work by early March.

As soon as I saw the doctor, I knew that he had some news for us and his expression told me that it wasn't going to be glad tidings. He spoke softly and gently for a change. I detected that this was going to be as difficult for him to tell as it was for us to hear.

"I'm really sorry, guys," he started, "but the scan indicates that the cancer has moved into your pelvis. All the evidence suggests that you have bone cancer."

Glancing at Carol, I noticed tears were rolling down her cheeks and into her lap. No sound accompanied her tears as she struggled to fight them back but I knew that for her, this was absolute devastation. I put my hand on her shoulder in support and asked Freidman the same question I always asked. "What is the next step?" I had come this far and was certainly not about to give up. He said that I should see the radiologist in a few days and discuss the appropriate treatment. Once again Freidman apologised for the news, saying, "Hang on in there, guys. We will get you through it." This was particularly aimed at Carol, who was clearly very distressed and thinking that we were fighting a losing battle. I, on the other hand, was not ready to concede defeat yet. We may be losing the battle but I was determined that we would win the war. I saw this as simply one more step I had to go through to beat this mighty foe.

---

I first saw the radiologist, Doctor Maloney, on 28th of January. I'd taken my bone and CAT scans with me for the appointment and he was on the other side of the room studying them in fine detail while we waited. He came over to the couch where the nurse had prepared me earlier, and started pressing around the area of the apparent cancer. He asked me a lot of questions like: "Have you ever broken your pelvis?" Which I hadn't, and; "Do you ever have any pain here?" Again, I assured him that I didn't. He said that the diagnosis bothered him as he would expect to find some discomfort in the general area associated with cancer. He led us across the room and showed us the bone scan on the viewing panel. He pointed out the white areas in my pelvis which, effectively, was evident across the whole of the left side of my pelvis.

"This is the area of concern," he told us. "I would

like to be a lot clearer about exactly what this is before we decide on any course of treatment."

I was quite surprised by this comment as I thought it had already been determined that it was cancer. However, he held out a ray of hope when he mentioned that the results of the scan actually said, "The findings are typical of either prostate carcinoma, metastatic to bone or of Paget's disease, but because of the patient's history, carcinoma of the prostate metastatic to bone is suspected." He told me that he wasn't ruling out the possibility of Paget's disease.

"Paget's disease?" I said in complete bewilderment. "What's that?" I was already thinking that this could be better news although I'd never heard of Paget's disease and didn't have any idea if it was going to be more or less of a problem than bone cancer. Maloney explained that it is a metabolic bone disease that involves bone destruction and re-growth, resulting in deformity. Apparently, it is indistinguishable from cancer on the bone scan. This would account for his questions about any previous break of my pelvis. He told me he wanted me to have some X-rays so that he had a clearer picture. I left his office and went immediately to the X-ray department as instructed. I was as keen as Maloney to find out what this might reveal.

I was completely bewildered; Maloney was looking into Paget's disease although I knew I'd never had a fractured pelvis at any time in my life. Once we returned home, I started my research about the disease. I needed to know more before I could get it clear in my mind. What I discovered made me slightly more optimistic but I was still unclear of my own position. However, I could now appreciate Maloney's reasoned approach. (For more information, I have set out a summary of my findings in Appendix C).

I now had the information I needed but felt no further forward in my knowledge of what was going on in my pelvis. I would simply have to wait for the expert view. Unfortunately, this was easier said than done. What we all hope is that experts are just that; Expert! When they come to a conclusion, you can be confident that they have made a correct diagnosis. But what happens when the experts disagree? I was about to find out.

A couple of days after my X-rays, I had a call from Maloney's office to say that he wanted me to have another bone scan. I was told that the hospital would call me to make an appointment. The message didn't convey the fact that I was about to enter a war zone. The phone rang again and this time it was a nurse from the Nuclear Medicine office asking if I could come in for the bone scan the next day. I confirmed that I could and the appointment was set for eight o clock in the morning.

Only a few minutes later the phone rang again and the voice at the other end identified itself as Doctor Steinberg. He was the head of Nuclear Medicine and responsible for interpreting the results of bone scans. He appeared somewhat grumpy but asked if I could come over to his office now. I said I could and that it would take me about twenty minutes. Wasting no time, I arrived at the office to find Doctor Steinberg waiting in Reception for me. This appeared slightly odd to me but I guessed that the department wasn't particularly busy that day. He showed me into his large, plush office. It was panelled in oak and grandly furnished with an imposing oak desk as the centre-piece. I knew that this was the 'inner sanctum' of Nuclear Medicine and not an area that many patients would normally see. Obviously, for some reason I was unaware of, I was getting special treatment. He looked me squarely in the eyes and said, "I'm not happy when my professional integrity is called into question." This comment took me so much by surprise that I looked behind me to see if someone had just entered the office behind me and Steinberg was addressing his remarks to him. No, no one was there. He must be talking to me. He was clearly looking for a response but I didn't have one. I had no idea what he was talking about. Eventually, I responded with the only thing that made any sense.

"I'm sure you're not," I concluded.

"Why do you think you need another bone scan?" he demanded.

Thankfully we were now on to easy questions and I said, "Because Doctor Maloney has told me to have one."

At this point it must have dawned on Steinberg that I had no idea what he was talking about and he set about explaining that he and Maloney had had a serious disagreement about the results of the first scan, with Steinberg saying that it was cancer and Maloney saying that the scan was unclear and it was more likely that I had Paget's disease. Finally, Maloney had ordered another scan which had obviously annoyed Steinberg. This was all very well but I was the piggy in the middle. As far as I was concerned, Steinberg's professional pride could go to hell. I needed the best opinion about what was happening in my pelvis and if it meant multiple bone scans, then so be it.

Soon I was back on the table but this time, Steinberg was doing the scan himself – minus my pads. After the scan was complete he told me to get dressed and wait in his office. I had just sat down when he came in waving the scan and saying, "I knew I was right." He led me to the viewing room and switched the light on the viewing box so that we could both see the results. He meticulously took me through what he was seeing on the scan and told me that his original diagnosis had been correct.

I was indignant. Rage was starting to build up inside me and at last it found a voice, "Well, it may be good news for you but it's bloody bad news for me, isn't it?"

He looked at me quite sympathetically and said, "Yes, I'm afraid it is and I'm sorry you were caught up in all this."

Well, at least he had apologised, but I felt really angry. Angry that Steinberg had been so unprofessional as to involve me in this fiasco. His dispute with Maloney was of no concern to me and I expected him to be doing whatever was best for me – not to involve himself in petty bickering about his professional integrity while I was going through hell, not knowing what lay ahead. As I left his office, I felt quite down for the first time. It felt to me like all hope was fading and I was facing a protracted period of suffering as the cancer ate deeper into my bones. Steinberg may have won his argument but I was the loser. My dismay didn't last for long though. As I drove home from the hospital I was already bouncing back. I wasn't going to let it get to me.

When I had first come to Houston, like most visitors, I had been to the Johnson Space Centre. The one thing that had fixed in my mind from that visit was the credo of those guys at mission control. 'Failure is not an option.' It proved to be such a powerful maxim during the fated Apollo 13 mission, when the team had brought the crew safely back to earth against all the odds. Clearly, we are all susceptible to failure, but I realised that what this adage really meant was that, by accepting it as an option, was to accept that the effort to succeed would likely be reduced. Positive mental attitude can move mountains and as long as I had any fight left in me, I was sure as hell going to use it. I knew I could pull through.

I turned my thinking to the next step in my war on this disease; a disease most people would rather refer to as the 'dreaded 'C' word' but to me the word came more easily. Cancer was proving itself to be a hostile foe - but it hadn't got me yet and failure was not an option.

# 13
## Paget's or Cancer. That is the Question

It was the end of January and Carol was persevering with the burden of changing my dressing four times a day. She had done an excellent job and my wound was nearly healed. Only a few more days would do it. She had been extremely depressed since day one, and living in a strange country, not knowing anyone and having to deal with my cancer on a daily basis was taking its toll. I would sometimes catch her crying for no apparent reason and it was hell for me to watch, knowing I could do nothing to help. I was the problem and she was determined to work through it with me but it was proving to be very difficult for her. I felt that she needed a break from my problems and me and urged her on several occasions to take a short holiday in the UK, where she could be with friends. She wouldn't hear of it, citing the need for my change of dressings as the reason. However, with this nearing the end, I had another try and suggested that I could manage for a week, while she relaxed for a while. She wasn't convinced by my argument so I tried a different tack. I was certain that she was so close to the problem that she couldn't get a proper perspective. At least if she was able to talk it through with people she trusted, it might help her to deal with it more readily. To emphasize my point, I told her a truth that had remained unspoken for a month. Her pain and anguish was pulling me down. I'd managed to be positive so far, but my concerns for her wellbeing were taking all my strength to deal with. I knew that she couldn't pretend to be happy, and nor did I want that, but I was hoping that in time she would learn to live with the situation and deal with each setback as it presented itself. The only way I could see that she could get a clearer perspective was to be away from me and the treatment, and talk it through with people who were less close to the problems. I knew this was bordering on emotional blackmail but I needed all my strength to fight the beast inside me, and I was finding it difficult to be strong for her at the same time.

She didn't immediately agree, later she said that maybe it would be a good idea if she were to get away for a few days. I took her at her word and within ten minutes I'd booked her a flight through the Internet. I hoped she didn't feel that I was pushing her away but I was sure the break would do us both some good. At present, she was worrying about me and I was worrying about her worrying about me. We needed some space.

As if by magic, the day before she was due to leave on her trip, my wound completed its healing process and so any concern Carol had had about me managing was removed. Now she could go without the guilt she was feeling about leaving me on my own.

That evening, a good friend of mine rang to say that he would be in Houston the following week. John and I had shared many drinks together, and at times we indulged to excess. However, mostly we were restrained, restricting our intake to no more that eight pints in a session. After asking how I was, he said, "How about downing a few pints when I'm over?" Although I hadn't lost the taste for the amber nectar, I was a bit reluctant.

## Please Leave The Seat Up

I told him that we could go for a drink but mine would be red wine as capacity was everything these days, and besides, the doctor had prescribed red wine for me so I felt duty bound to take my medicine.

The day after Carol left for the UK, Maloney rang and asked me to call into his office. He now had the results of the second bone scan, which according to Steinberg was conclusive. But still Maloney was unconvinced, or at least he wasn't prepared to accept it without wanting more evidence. He advised me that he wanted me to have a bone biopsy, which would determine once and for all whether cancer was present. I didn't know what a bone biopsy involved but the biopsy of my prostate was still a relatively fresh recollection and I knew that it wasn't a pleasant experience. I could only hope the bone biopsy would be less painful but somehow I doubted it. The doctor told me that the hospital would contact me with an appointment so I went home and phoned Carol with the news. She was lifted by this new step, believing that once again there was hope. This was characteristic of how she treated all the news, seeing a ray of hope as positive and a setback as extremely negative, which led to her riding an emotional roller coaster. I feared for her if the results proved to be another disappointment, as this would send her crashing down into the depths of despair once again. I was much calmer about this, treating it as simply another piece of news until such time as we had a definitive diagnosis and clear understanding of things. Carol now had a new dilemma: She was concerned that she wasn't going to be with me when they carried out the procedure. I promised her that I wouldn't commit to an appointment until she got back to the US. As it turned out, the first appointment they offered was on 10th February, two days after Carol's return. This was perfect, especially as I preferred not to have to wait for too long. The uncertainty was really getting to both of us.

By the fifth day of Carol's holiday, I was starting to miss her. After all, we had spent almost every waking moment together since early December, and I'd come to rely on her for everything. Catering for myself wasn't difficult, as Carol had prepared meals for every day that she expected to be away. All I had to do was follow the detailed instruction she had left. Mind you, my culinary skills are such that even following instructions on the pack is no guarantee for a gastronomic success. On a previous occasion I had promised Carol that I would cook dinner. She was suspicious and more than a bit concerned but when I told her it would be chilli-con-carne from a pack, and a tin of Uncle Ben's rice, she felt that even I couldn't mess it up. Wrong! We ended up with ratatouille and rice. I'd opened the wrong packet. Still, I was getting by okay and although the food always managed to taste a little strange, it kept me alive and free from hunger. I now know that if I need an effective weight-loss diet, I should start cooking for myself. It is so tasteless that I can only eat enough of it to sustain life. It's certainly not 'eating for pleasure'.

Apart from the cooking, I did miss her. Although her constant checking to see if I was OK had occasionally got on my nerves sometimes, I now wished she was back with me, getting on my nerves again. I could tell from her phone calls that the break was doing her some good and I never shared my thoughts with her, not wishing to unsettle her, but I was gladdened to hear that she was so keen to get back home with me. The time passed soon enough and I was delighted when she returned. Now we could face the bone biopsy together, hopefully after a good meal for a change.

We arrived at the hospital in plenty of time for our eight o'clock appointment. A nurse got me sorted out with a gown and onto a hospital trolley. She took us through the process in fine detail, answering any questions that we had. I was to have a 'CAT scan assisted bone biopsy', which meant that I would be in the scanner while the surgeon used the CAT scan image to correctly position his instruments for the procedure. I would have a local anaesthetic and when I was groggy, I would be placed under the machine while he plunged a long, hollow, large diameter needle into my stomach and through onto my pelvic bone. He would reposition it as necessary until he was satisfied that it was exactly in the right place and then remove a piece of bone from my pelvis.

I was glad to hear that I would be groggy during the process but felt that a full bottle of Scotch might help me a whole lot more in the groggy stakes. Apparently, that wasn't on their approved list of anaesthesia so we stuck to the more traditional method. I hoped they were planning to use plenty of it. It's not that I'm a coward – well, actually I am - but it sounded pretty awful. As it turned out it wasn't anything like I was expecting - it was much, much worse.

The surgeon gave me a warm friendly smile as he started to insert the needle. I was barely conscious but became aware of some pain as he pushed the needle further and further through the overly adequate layers of flesh and fat, delving ever closer to my pelvic bone. Several times I felt him repositioning the needle and was willing him to get it over with. Finally, he had the position he needed and now he was going to take the sample. It hadn't occurred to me exactly how this would be done but I was about to find out. The first clue was when he requested a hammer from his nurse.

He proceeded to hammer away, apparently on the needle, trying to knock a piece of bone free from the pelvis. I'm sure that as you read this you're trying to imagine what this would be like. Well, you cannot imagine it and hopefully you will never need to find out. But as I lay there in my semi-comatose state, wishing now that I'd insisted on the whisky, I became aware of every inch of my skeleton as the hammer blows reverberated throughout my body. It wasn't excruciatingly painful but it was an experience that I would rather have left undiscovered. Unfortunately, the surgeon was having some trouble shifting the bone and the hammering went on for what seemed like a lifetime. Finally, he got a piece of bone free and concluded the process. It had only taken about fifteen minutes but, just like banging your head against a brick wall, it was really good when it stopped.

I was wheeled away to a recovery room to allow the anaesthetic to wear off before being discharged. I'd obviously had a big dose of the stuff as I didn't come

# Please Leave The Seat Up

round until two in the afternoon. Even then I was extremely wobbly. Walking was definitely still not part of my skill set. Thankfully, the nurse helped me into a wheelchair and pushed me to the hospital entrance where she helped me into the car for my journey home. The next day, after the anaesthetic had worn off, I was expecting to be in some pain but actually, I had only few after effects and within a couple of days, all discomfort had gone: only the nightmare of the hammering of my skeleton remained to haunt me.

A week later we returned to Maloney's office for a review of the bone biopsy. At last this was a good news day. He told us that the biopsy had revealed no trace of cancer in the pelvis. He was now convinced that what we were looking at in the previous scans was indeed Paget's disease. However, he suggested that I needed to have a PSA and a PAP test, to be absolutely certain. I think this was for our benefit rather than his.

He told me that in his opinion I wasn't ready for the radiation treatment just yet as I was still struggling to control my bladder. He wanted me to improve the control before we got the radiation treatment underway. He made us an appointment to see him again on 19th March to review my readiness and requested that I have the tests one week prior to the appointment, so that we could review those results at the same time.

When we were driving home I was feeling quite elated but Carol was more subdued. She was hoping for a definitive result but felt that having two more tests was another postponement of the certainty we were looking for. I, on the other hand, felt that we already had the certainty we needed. If no cancer had been found in the bone sample, what more proof did we need? Rather than worry about the results of the two additional tests, my only task for the next month was going to be to concentrate on getting my bladder control improved enough to start the radiation treatment. However, I did take a few minutes to find out what a PAP test was likely to reveal. I was already familiar with the PSA (or Prostate Specific Antigen) test was and expected the reading to be less than 0.1. (For information I have included a summary of information on PAP in Appendix D).

---

During the first week of March I attended a routine visit to Freidman. He asked for a PSA test and told me that he was extremely pleased with my progress, especially my bladder control. I was making a concerted effort with my Keygel's, which was now starting to produce some good results. Most of the time I was able to get to a toilet in time to have normal bodily functions, although coughing, sneezing, climbing, bending and stretching all presented a constant challenge to me. He said he didn't need to see me again for three months. I felt this was a big step forward: Another good day – or so I thought.

As I was emptying my bladder at about five o clock that evening, I noticed that my urine looked pink. I mentioned it to Carol and she produced a jar asking me to use it the next time I needed to go, so that we could look at it a bit more closely. About an hour later I picked up the jar and started to pee. There was no need for close inspection any more. I was urinating neat blood; red and frothy. I was so concerned: my initial thoughts were that this was truly serious and the cancer was taking over. For the first time I had visions of my life coming to an early and abrupt end. Once again, we were heading to the ER for another $75 contribution to my treatment. We were both extremely worried and in an attempt to lighten our mood a little I suggested to Carol that this might be part of the effects of my hormone treatment. I pointed out that I now had so many female hormones inside me that this could be the start of my menstruation cycle. We both laughed but it didn't hide our fear. Fortunately, it turned out to be a bladder infection. The hospital doctor advised me to see Freidman the next morning. This was becoming a habit.

When I saw Freidman the next day I reminded him that every time he gave me good news, I ended up back in his office the next day with a new problem. I don't think he found that particularly amusing. He said that he was happy with the diagnosis and treatment from the hospital and that I only needed to see him again if it didn't clear up in a few days. He also had some more good news for me. The PSA which had been carried out the day before, showed a reading of <1 which means no trace of cancer. I was delighted and almost glad that I'd needed to go back and see him so soon. I knew now that the PSA & PSP tests due the following week were going to give the desired results and we would be clear for my radiation treatment.

One of the more positive side effects of the bladder

infection was that I now had complete bladder control. In fact, for a couple of days I hardly passed water at all, which made me feel almost normal again. Unfortunately, as the infection cleared, my lack of bladder control was demanding my full attention once again and I was back to my regular round of Keygels and Paddy Pads.

## 14
## Eradication

The meeting with Doctor Maloney on 19th March turned out to be a most memorable occasion as well as an important milestone in my progress. We finally got confirmation that as far as could be determined through tests, no cancer was present in my pelvis. This now left the way clear for us to move forward with the radiation stage of my treatment, which was necessary to completely eradicate the traces of cancerous cells in the area of my prostate left after the operation.

Carol and I were both delighted and relieved with the news and I asked the doctor, out of interest, what treatment would have been required if it had been confirmed as bone cancer. He didn't have a definitive answer but felt that most likely it would have been palliative care. Clearly, he wouldn't have gone ahead with the radiation, seeing no benefit in putting me through the side effects whilst losing the battle to control the disease. A sobering thought and one I'm glad he hadn't shared with us earlier.

Maloney decided on a treatment regime of 32 sessions of 'external radiation therapy to the pelvic bed'. This was due to take place over a seven-week period on each weekday, giving me weekends off for good behaviour. These "off days" were designed to give my body a much-needed rest and as benign cells recover more quickly than malignant cells, more of the benign cells survive with "off days."

The doctor handed me over to his nurse who meticulously described the dos and don'ts that I should follow for the duration of my treatment. Basically, I needed to avoid washing the target marks off when I bathed and not to expose my area of treatment to direct sunlight for extended periods. Given that the area was only inches above my penis I was guessing that she thought I was some sort of weirdo nudist or phantom flasher in my spare time.

She then talked through the potential side effects of the treatment with me. I already knew what they were, but she told me again all the same, reading strictly from her list and leaving nothing out. They included bladder irritation and more frequent urination, sometime leading to poor bladder control. (What a blow: Just when I was starting to get it sorted). In addition, irritation of the rectum, bleeding and diarrhoea are possibilities, together with increased fatigue as I work through the treatment. The area for radiation can be sore with skin irritation, and may need treatment. Finally, she advised that this would have an adverse effect on my potency.

"Oh no!" I exclaimed, in mock surprise and my voice filled with anguish.

She looked at me with concern, not sure how she should respond to my apparent distress.

"First they took away my prostate without being able to spare the nerves, leaving me completely impotent. Next they put me on a course of hormone treatment which has chemically castrated me, and now you tell me that the radiation treatment will cause impotency: How much more impotent do you think I can get and how will it manifest itself?"

The nurse continued to stare at me, but this time in astonishment. I knew that I'd gone too far. Americans are not big on irony and she appeared relieved after I told her I was only teasing.

I attended the hospital on 25th March for yet another CAT scan, but this time it was so that the radiation technologist could see how my internal organs in that area were configured. From this information, she was able to measure and mark the 'target' area with indelible pen. By the time I left the hospital, I looked like a human target with crosses on my front and both sides. My first session of treatment was scheduled for two days later.

The routine for the treatment was that I would lie on a bed, which was then raised to about five feet from the ground, with the radiation machine hovering just above me. Lead-shielding blocks were placed at the radiation beam aperture to protect non-cancerous tissue when the radiation was applied and to produce a more precise beam. When everything was ready, the technician called, "Take aim – fire." (He didn't really but there were occasions when I was sure I heard someone calling it out in my head). I was then subjected to high energy X-rays from the linear accelerator. This process, called three-dimensional conformal therapy, also reduced the risk of side effects.

## Brian Turner

Once a week during the treatment, I saw the doctor and he would ask about my progress. His questions were always the same and I became familiar with what he was going to say:

"How is your flow of urine?"

"How is the pressure? Do you have a good steady stream?"

"Do you have any signs of blood present in your urine?"

"How frequently are you having your bowels open?"

"What is the texture like?" (Ugghh! What an awful question.)

"Are you experiencing any pain, associated with your toilet actions?"

"Are you experiencing any rectal bleeding?"

Obviously, he was anticipating some problems and his questions were an indication that they may be extremely unpleasant. Every week I was glad to report that everything was OK and I started to feel that it was all a bit of a breeze – until week five. Then things started to change. Slowly at first, but before long my bowels and bladder had taken on a mind of their own. I was finding it difficult to leave the house for any length of time, for fear of being caught short. It was all highly unpredictable and caught me out on a number of occasions. There's more than one restaurant in Houston, which wouldn't welcome me back in a hurry. Well, not without a bucket and shovel anyway.

The 12th May marked the point exactly nine months since I'd moved to America. It was also the date of my final radiation treatment. I asked Carol to bake a cake for the staff at the centre who had all been so kind and exceptional in their bedside manner. After being zapped for the last time, I saw the doctor for his normal round of questions, although by now, I wasn't saying no to all of them. I was having a lot of problems with what he euphemistically referred to as 'rectal urgency'. He told me that things should start to improve slowly and asked me to see him again in six weeks to check on progress. I was so relieved that the treatment was over. It was never painful or unpleasant, but I wanted my bowels and bladder back to normal. I wasn't to know it then, but that process was going to take quite a time.

As I left the hospital, I handed the team the cake and a card on which I'd written, "It's been great to see you all every day, but I hope never to see any of you again."

The following day I went back to the hospital for my second injection of Lupron. After the nurse had 'stuck' me in the hip, I asked if I was going to see Freidman.

"No," she replied, a bit surprised by my question.

"When should I see him again, then?" I asked.

"I expect he'll want to catch up with you again in about six months, just to see how things are going."

As I walked from the hospital to my car I felt empty and despondent. It was a feeling I rarely get and couldn't understand why I felt it now. And then it hit me. Tomorrow, for the first day in many months, I didn't have to go to the hospital. In fact, I didn't even have any appointments scheduled. I guess this was a sign that things were going well, but it didn't feel good. It felt, well ---- strange. In a mild attack of panic, I started to mull over the many unanswered questions I had. They hadn't been a concern to me all the time I was going to the hospital regularly and my questions remained unasked, but suddenly I was out of the loop and now they would remain unanswered, at least for a while, and I didn't know how to deal with them.

"Am I clear of cancer?"

"Do I need any further treatment?"

"What checks will I need in the future?"

"Is there anything that can be done about my impotency?"

It appeared that everything had suddenly come to an end and I was left in the cold. (Metaphorically, you understand. In the literal sense, one is never cold in Houston). I felt alone, abandoned. For the first time since it all began, I WAS SCARED

## 15
## 'Ow's it Going?

I once worked for a big, earthy Yorkshireman, who would often say to his staff, "'ow's it goin' then?" It sounded like a general enquiry about one's health but, as people who worked for him soon found out, this apparently casual enquiry was a thinly disguised euphemism for, 'sit down and spill your guts. Tell me everything you know, starting from the beginning and leaving nothing out. More precisely, feel free to dish the dirt on your friends and colleagues, so that I will have ammunition against them for the future, should I need it. My intention here however, is merely to give an update on progress following the radiation treatment.

I kept my appointment with Maloney at the end of June. I was disappointed that I was making slower progress than I'd hoped. I hadn't been prepared for the fact that things could get worse after the treatment had ended, but that's exactly what happened. I suffered badly from fatigue, sometimes falling asleep without warning. Exercise was necessary but the fatigue sapped my stamina and I appeared to get slower and more tired with each passing day. Over the next few weeks I put on all the weight I lost before the operation. Carrying extra weight is not particularly helpful when you need to manage your bladder.

One additional side effect of the hormone and radiation treatments started to build in early June. I began to feel guilty about not being at work, although I was also anxious about the prospect of going back. My previous enthusiasm to operate with the movers and shakers wasn't there. My confidence had taken a tumble and my emotions were always hovering just below the surface. I would laugh uncontrollably about the slightest thing or find myself weeping mercilessly at anything that was a little sad. I couldn't seem to 'get a grip' and I started to panic.

I went along to see Doctor Epstein and shared my concerns with him. He smiled as I went through a litany of symptoms. I read from a list I'd prepared for the meeting as forgetfulness was one of the problems. When I got to the end of my list, he said, "At last!"

"At last, what?" I queried, not knowing what he meant.

"At last you admit to having some problems. Throughout the whole of the treatment, I was thinking that you were some kind of superman. Whenever I saw you, you told me you were great and things were all going well. I have marvelled at your fortitude and resolve; your determination to get through it come what may. But you are allowed to be ill, you know. You are allowed to feel low and sad on occasions, like the rest of us mere mortals."

I took his point. In my efforts to deal with this invasive disease, I'd wanted to stay positive and convinced myself that everything was fine. In fact, most of the time it was, but dealing with the treatment was proving to be a whole lot more difficult than dealing with cancer. I was well on the road to recovery and it was now time to be more relaxed. I wasn't fighting the cancer head-on anymore and I could afford to allow the healing process to takes its course, even though it might be slow and tiring at times. Realising by now that this was going to be a slow process, I raised the issue of my return to work with my boss and the HR manager. They were still playing things very low key, happy to wait until I was ready. We discussed a number of options for the future once I was fully recovered. One of the suggestions made - very gingerly so as not to hurt my feelings I suspect - was that I put myself forward for early retirement on medical grounds. I had always planned to retire early at around 55 but this would bring the date forward by two years. I gave it some thought and concluded that as my life expectancy had potentially taken a hit, Carol and I should seize the chance. My pension would be sufficient and I now knew that spending our time together was far more important than any money. This became an easy decision as it was a good opportunity and I told my boss I would like to accept it.

In a relatively short period, we unwound our life in the US and returned to the UK, but not before we took a short holiday in Hawaii. We hadn't planned it but we had to vacate our house two weeks before we were due to leave Houston. A few days before we were to become homeless I said to Carol, "We will need to stay in a hotel for a couple of weeks, but why does it have to be in Houston"? She asked where I had in mind. "How about Hawaii"? I reasoned that although it was 6 hours flying time away, we were probably the closest we would ever be and it would be a good opportunity to see a place most people only dream of. And so it was that on 20th September we flew off to our own piece of the paradise island of Maui. It was a great place to relax and a wonderful ending to our American experience.

We arrived back in the UK on 1st October 2003 at 07.00. It was a cold, grey, misty morning and already Hawaii seemed to be a million miles away. However, we really enjoyed catching up with all our friends and family who had been so supportive of us during the past twelve months. Although we had to wait another month before our furniture arrived, we did move back in to our house, sitting on deck chairs and sleeping on a put-you-up; but we were home.

My first task on our return was to get myself registered with a GP. I was quite concerned that with my recent problems it may prove to be difficult. Fortunately, I found one very close by who appeared to be happy to take me on and he became quite fascinated as I talked through my recent medical history. He ventured the suggestion that going to America had probably saved my life. I was certainly in agreement with that sentiment. When we had finished he said, "It sounds like you know more about prostate cancer than I do." I hoped he was joking.

He sorted through my list of drugs and told me that he would have to find alternatives to some as they were exclusive to the US market, but he soon had me fixed up with what I needed and I became a regular visitor to our local chemist, emerging from the shop, clutching hold of my bag of goodies every month. However, my confidence that my treatment would continue with a seamless change was soon to be tested. During a routine visit to the surgery in November, I asked when my PSA test was due. The doctor gave me a blank look and shrugged, as if to say, *why are you asking me?* I told him that according to my records, my next test was imminent. He agreed to do it, but I realised that I was now going to have to take responsibility to ensure I got the tests and treatment I needed. This was not going to be the automatic process it had been in the US. A few weeks later I requested that I be referred to an urologist. Again, my GP was puzzled at the request and I had to insist that I needed my cancer to be closely monitored by an expert, at least for the time I continued with the hormone therapy. I started to believe that his earlier comment about his knowledge of prostate cancer had not been a joke after all. He made a referral and a couple of weeks later I received a letter from the hospital to inform me that there was a 27 week wait before I would get onto the waiting list. – Welcome Home!

There were many things we missed about America apart from the fabulous sunny weather of the Gulf coast region. They were mainly little things, like sitting outside Starbucks with tall Latte, watching the world go by, or the excellent service one gets in any shop, restaurant or garage. However, the thing I miss the most are public toilets. We had been used to these facilities everywhere, grocery stores, hobby stores, gas stations, parks and even in the pharmacy. I hadn't thought of it before but these facilities are sadly lacking from the UK infrastructure and I now have to search them out and plan journeys far more carefully. A car journey of more than two hours has to include a stop at a *Little Chef* or a Motorway service area: And a trip across London on the underground is a challenge; not one to be undertaken lightly and never even considered during the rush hour.

Throughout my illness and the various treatments, I have spent many hours surfing the Internet in order to get more information about the beast that was trying to kill me. Fortunately, the electronic age has caused such an enormous amount to be written and stored on the web that I was able to get up to speed very quickly, once I put my mind to it. Unfortunately, that was mainly after I'd had the operation. If I had to go through it again, I would make the educational leap a lot earlier.

One of the things, which I overlooked in the early stages, either through my lack of knowledge or an overly optimistic view of life, was to make contact with a support group. Included amongst the support groups for all types of cancer are those for cancer of the prostate. These usually consist of sufferers and survivors as well as health experts, who provide help, support and advice from the time cancer is diagnosed, right through the treatment and recovery phase and beyond. Through my ignorance, Carol and I trod the path alone, and sometimes it was a lonely place to be. I often wonder now what useful tips and advice I might have obtained if I'd linked up with a group from the outset. I wonder if they have discovered *my device* and if not, would they welcome the information. I know for sure that in those difficult days, I would have been delighted for someone to enlighten me. As it was, it sometimes felt like I was the only man who ever had to tackle such issues. On arrival back in the UK, I looked up support groups for my area, only now I was keen to be providing support to others, rather than being in need of it. Through this effort, I made contact with one of the prostate charities and soon signed myself up to help. However, I was a man on a mission and felt that this wasn't enough. I needed to help educate people and raise awareness; to spread the word more widely. During November and December I held three seminars on 'Caring for the Prostate' for my company. These went extremely well and were attended by both men and women. Interestingly, it was the women asked the most interesting and probing questions. I have since been asked to speak at several more seminars in 2004, both for the company and to external organisations and I am looking forward to them.

---

The side effects during the first six months of my treatment were so varied that I was never quite sure what to expect next. Apart from all those I've mentioned earlier, I experienced drying of the skin around and in my ears and on my face, drying of my hair, to the extent that it felt like straw. I treated both of these with health products and eventually things returned to normal, although during one visit to the hairdresser, the lady cutting my hair said, "Your hair and skin are so dry; I would like you to try and use some moisturisers." I agreed that they were dry, but assured her that I was on the case. Insistent in making her point, she pushed a little harder saying that I should change to a different product, as the one I was using didn't appear to be working. This in-your-face approach is quite common in the US but I think the hairdresser wished she hadn't mentioned it when I replied; "The problem is caused by my cancer treatment." She was silent for a few seconds and then said, almost in a whisper, "I'm so sorry." Of course, there was no need for her to be sorry and I hadn't intended to shock her or make her feel embarrassed. I was only trying to explain the problem but once again, the mention of cancer got the same reaction as exploding a hand grenade.

I have noticed that my body hair has almost completely disappeared. My chest and underarms are bald and my arms and legs are heading the same way. Luckily, the 'straw' on my head is as strong as ever and the barber always comments on it when I go for a re-thatch. My breasts have also developed, although with the rest of my body fat competing for space, I'm not sure they notice too much. I'm guessing that these changes are due to the upset of hormonal balance within my body as I now have more female than male hormones. However, I still manage to resist the temptation to go shopping for more shoes, although I would be happy for a night out with the girls once in a while.

I have often heard people use the phrase *cancer survivor*, as in; *I am a cancer survivor of seven years.* I always thought it was a trite and very American thing to say. After all, we all get ill but we never say, "I'm a measles survivor of twenty-two years," or "a 'flu survivor of six years." Well that's how I felt a year ago. Now, I have a different view. It's been twelve months since my operation and I'm doing well. I have hopefully completed all the major treatment I need, although I still have to continue with the jabs and pills of the hormone therapy for another two years. And I will need regular checks for many years to come, to ensure that the cancer cells aren't gathering again to do battle with this particular foe. If they do, I will be more than ready to fight again.

Life is not back to normal: In fact life will never be quite the same again. Not that it's worse, or better for that matter. However, it is different and I've learned to make the most of every moment as if it were my last. Work, which has always been such a vital part of my life and my motivation, has taken a lower order of importance and I am looking forward to *officially* retiring in February. I have missed the cut and thrust of business during my time away although it doesn't hold quite the same excitement for me as it once did. Priorities have taken on a different order and the things that really matter are those I have always taken for granted or never quite got round to doing: Like spending time with my friends and family or taking in the sights and sounds of the natural beauty that surround us all.

Prior to leaving America I saw a TV programme about the life of Lance Armstrong. Lance is best known for his achievement of winning the Tour de France cycle race five times in consecutive years[13], including 2003. What many people don't know about him is that seven years earlier he was diagnosed with testicular cancer. His offending testicle was immediately removed by

---

[13] He has subsequently won twice more before retiring after the 2005 Tour de France, making him a 7 times champion.

surgery, but within a few days, the doctors discovered that the cancer had also planted itself around his brain. Within three weeks, he underwent an extremely difficult operation to remove the tumour, followed by a long period of chemotherapy. It took him more than a year to recover from the treatment but his determination and guts to fight back against the odds was impressive against any measure. To win his first Tour de France the following year was simply astounding.

I have always been a positive person and have managed to stay strong through my illness, but Lance has shown us all the way through such a trauma. This gives me great hope for my own future, as I am also a fighter and determined to pull myself back up; to face new challenges the way I have faced them before; and to win. My time may not be spent in the same way as it has been previously but my enthusiasm to succeed will always be there. I will find new ways to make a contribution and whatever it takes; I will be pleased to have had the opportunity. Lance Armstrong has achieved so much in his cycling career and to take five wins at the Tour de France is a triumph, which understandably makes him beam with pride. However, in his interview he said that although winning the races had been extremely satisfying, his biggest achievement and the one of which he was most proud was beating cancer.

As I reflect on all that has happened since I first went to work in America, I realise that everything has conspired in my favour, making an awful and potentially life-threatening situation, both treatable and curable. Luck was on my side when I was posted there and it continued to play a role throughout the treatment. It is a sure thing that if I hadn't gone to the US, I wouldn't have discovered the disease until it was incurable and that makes me smile – frequently. Like Lance, I too am pleased to be able to say, "I am a cancer survivor".

# 16

# The Last Word

Writing this book was a cathartic exercise and kept me occupied through the various stages of my treatment. After completing it, I had intended to get it published but life started to get quite busy. The manuscript got put in the draw and forgotten. From time-to-time I would let people read it if they had a particular interest and they would usually encourage me to get on and publish. However, though my experience of the disease, I learned that doing the things that matter most to me and my wife is more important than anything else; so we went about moving house, spending time with friends and family and generally moving on. The book stayed in the draw.

Since returning to the UK I have regularly had my PSA tested as a precaution and the results always showed that the cancer was in remission. I was beginning to think that I could condemn the experience of the cancer to the past and looked forward to being taken off the hormone treatment very soon. Then, during a routine test in mid July 2005 my PSA was recorded at 56. As it was so high, I thought this must be a mistake and asked the doctor for a re-test. Two weeks later the reading was up to 87. Since then, with a change of drugs the reading is back down at 2 but the cancer has metastasised[14] to my liver and once again I have to do battle with this foe. But so far, I'm still standing and still smiling.

---

[14] To be transmitted or transferred by metastasis

# Appendix A

Useful questions for the Doctor upon being diagnosed with prostate cancer

- What do the results mean?
- How advanced is the cancer?
- How serious is my case in light of my general health conditions?
- What if the cancer has spread beyond my prostate? Is it still curable?
- What treatments are available and how effective are they for my particular case?
- What treatment do you recommend? What are the risks involved?
- What are the physical and emotional side effects of each treatment, and how are they managed?
- How much time can we take to make a treatment decision?
- Is it appropriate to obtain a second opinion? (This is commonplace in the US system.)
- Are there any dietary recommendations or restrictions before, during and after treatment?
- If an operation is required, how long will be necessary for the stay in hospital and the recovery?
- Are there informational brochures, books, video or audiotapes that we should obtain?
- Where can we find information about support groups?
- How can we find out about alternative medicines?
- What do we do next?

# Appendix B

# The TMN ranking system

The ranking table is set out below as an indication of how this works.

## *Tumour rating*

*T0: There is no evidence of a tumour.*

*T1: Primary tumours cannot be detected with a DRE or TRUS.*

*T2: The tumour is confined within the prostate and is detectable with DRE and TRUS.*

*T3: The tumour extends through the capsule of the prostate. This is more dangerous than if it were contained within the prostate.*

*T4: The tumour has invaded other organs.*

## *Node rating*

*N0: There is no lymph node involvement.*

*NX: The lymph nodes have not been assessed.*

*N1: The cancer can be found in one node in the area of the prostate.*

*N2: The cancer extends to multiple nodes.*

*N3: The cancer can be found in a mass not attached to the tumour.*

*N4: The cancer extends to multiple nodes in other parts*

*of the body.*

## Metastasis rating

*M-0: Metastasis is not detectable.*

*MX: Metastasis has not been assessed.*

*M1a: Evidence of the metastasis can be determined.*

*M1b: A single metastasis is located in a single site.*

*M1c: Multiple metastases are found in a single site.*

*M1d: Multiple metastases are found in multiple sites.*


*"Although the 'T' can readily be determined through a biopsy, at this stage the 'N' and 'M' are largely deduced rather than firmly established. Positive determination is made when the pathologist is able to study the prostate after it has been removed from the body."*

## Appendix C

## Paget's disease

The following explanation is a summary of the information I elicited from a number of different Internet sites.

*The cause of Paget's disease is unknown. It occurs worldwide, but is more common in Europe, Australia, and New Zealand. The disease is characterized by excessive breakdown of bone tissue, followed by abnormal bone formation. The new bone is structurally enlarged, but weakened and filled with new blood vessels. The disease may localise to one or two areas within the skeleton, or become widespread. It more commonly occurs after a fracture but can occur naturally, without any apparent reason. Frequently, it occurs in the pelvis, femur, tibia, vertebrae and clavicle.*

### *Symptoms*

- *Bone pain (may be severe and persistent)*
- *Joint pain or stiffness*
- *Headache*
- *Bowing of the legs*
- *Warmth of skin overlying affected bone*
- *Fracture*
- *Neck pain*
- *Reduced height*
- *Hearing loss*

## Please Leave The Seat Up

*Most patients have no symptoms. Localised Paget's disease requires no treatment, if there are no symptoms and no evidence of active disease. Orthopaedic surgery may be required to correct a specific deformity in severe cases.*

# Appendix D

# PAP test

From the Internet I learned that *PAP is a blood test that measures prostatic acid phosphatase (an enzyme found primarily in the prostate gland and semen) to determine the health of the prostate gland. Prostate dysfunction results in the release of PAP into the blood. It is carried out to determine the presence of prostate cancer, an abnormality of the prostate gland, or to follow the response of prostate cancer to treatment.*

Abnormal PAP values can be obtained for many reasons, the most common of which include:

- *Prostate cancer*
- *Prostate cancer that has spread outside the prostate (particularly to bone)*
- *Paget's disease (bones become thicker and softer)*
- *Infection (usually severe)*
- *Prostatitis*

ISBN 1412095297